LIFE WITH AURA

LIFE WITH AURA

Tibetan Shamanic Interpretation of the Aura

Patricia Pattie Pellicciotti

Foreword by Alfredo Lissoni

Author photo by Paolo Meyer

Cover Design and Graphics by David Garvin

Library of Congress Control Number: 2012913879
ISBN: Hardcover   978-1-4771-5381-9
              Softcover   978-1-4771-5380-2
              Ebook   978-1-4771-5382-6

www.Auraology.com
USA: Telephone: +1-832-884-1477
Fax: +1-530-364-8077
First Edition: *Convivere Con L'Aura* © Patricia M. Pellicciotti, 2000
Second Italian Edition: *Iniziazione alla lettura dell'Aura* © 2004 Edizione Mediterranee
English Edition: *Life with Aura* © Patricia M. Pellicciotti, 2012

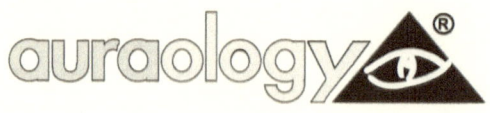

For Fun and for Real

This book was printed in the United States of America.

To order additional copies of this book, contact:
Xlibris Corporation
1-888-795-4274
www.Xlibris.com
Orders@Xlibris.com
119339

Contents

Part of the Proceeds is donated to charitable organizations that are near and dear to Patricia Pellicciotti's heart.

"If you want to learn all aspects of aura perception and diagnostics, your personal intuitive method, through the eyes of a Mystic: how to attain these heights, to emerge spiritually, then read this book from the life's experience of the author of over 40 years of research and practice."

Vivo Milano

"Many books about the Aura have been written, but this volume has a unique particularity: it explores the spell binding argument from the Tibetan Shaman point of view, little known to us outside the world of the Tibetan culture. The author, Patricia Pellicciotti, noted clairvoyant and prognostic, Italian-American from New York, is engaged in parapsychology and alternative medicine, Shaman healing and energy equilibrium. This volume speaks about her experience as a clairvoyant and receptor of transcendental messages and faith healing through the metaphysical. It describes all the techniques and secrets in a simple, concise and doable approach for the study, awareness and understanding necessary to familiarize you—for the first time-with all the mysteries surrounding this theme and gives you command of your mystical AURA"

MAGIC WORLD Magazine, Dario Spada, book critic

"Reading Aura Reading Initiation is like a refreshing dive into a natural spring. It's inspirational, simple to follow and rich."

Institute of Human Science & Jasmine Magazine,
Founder, Editor

Dedication

I dedicate this work to all my family, friends, and clients.

I wish to thank them for giving me the encouragement and feedback necessary to hone in on and refine my skills.

Given that life is a continuous learning cycle, I wish to remember those with whom I've had minimal success as a psychological consultant. I thank them for keeping me on my toes and keeping me humble. Through them I remain constantly aware that we are not all things to all people. To those I wish that universal energy and prayers will some day penetrate and take hold and produce positive effects.

I thank Italy for giving me an additional forum to perform God's work. I also thank the United States for giving me the universal school of preparation and experience and freedom to flourish.

Above all, I dedicate this work to God, in all His/Her divinities, whatever His/Her names are.

To the Supreme Entities, that all the fires of anger might be transformed and become fires of love.

Thank you for your unconditional love, Mom and Dad, I was really lucky to have been born to you both. Wish you were still with us to see the fruits of your hard labor.

Foreword

Patricia Pellicciotti, other than having a profound knowledge of the paranormal world and mediumship, is herself a mystic and shaman. Her background completely and thoroughly emerges in this book, in that it distinguishes itself with explicit clarity and with rich documentation.

The theme of this book is the Aura, the reality of which was at one time denied but is now growing again in acceptance and acknowledgment in many Occidental academic environments. The author presents this discussion through a precise excursus that is historical and geographical, passing from traditional India to Tibet to European and American experiments conducted over the last three centuries.

But Patricia Pellicciotti goes well beyond that, from her revelation of new frontiers related to more recent archaeological discoveries to that of the shamanic tradition and to the other extreme of new scientific documentation delineated with *mille metric* precision. She offers an extremely complete image of the Aura, replete with knowledge of that which the Russian scholars of the '70s called "the energetic soul of man."

And this is only the beginning. The volume explains, comprehensibly and in detail, how to visualize the Aura and how to interpret it based on color tones and musical chords (connecting our state of mind with our state of health), which helps explain the interventions necessary to obtain a healthy psychophysical state through the technique of meditation and Tibetan rituals. All are illustrated with simple exercises that anyone can do. If that is not enough, Patricia Pellicciotti has undergone a series of scientific experiments that test her psychic energy; the results are displayed and delineated at the end of the book.

As the editor of one of the principal publications in this field, and one who has worked in this arena for years, rarely have I seen among the vast and sometimes chaotic editions of the mysterious, a publication so distinguished and clearly factual and well-stated. Patricia Pellicciotti does so not only via validated data, but also with significant documentation.

The author obviously possesses a profound and studious *cognoscente*—the fruit of years of experience in research and practice—absolutely not to be missed. We will certainly hear about her again.

Alfred Lissoni
Editor in chief, *The Magazine: Knowledge Beyond*, Milan, Italy
Italian Title: *Oltre La Conoscenza*

Preface: The Auraology Approach to Self-Healing

Wherever there is life there is an Aura. Simply, the Aura sustains our life and surrounds the very subtle mind of the heart. The Aura forms a protective shield around our body, a sort of energetic immune system that defends us or guards us from all negative energies and diseases. This spiritual immune system or antibody maintains our daily needs and existence and induces our pathological resistance. In good health, the great force of these radiations of antibodies counteract germs and bacteria that are inimical to physical health. In other words, you could look at the Aura as the great inoculation from the sky. In sickness, these Aura emanations do not so easily eliminate disease germs. As a result, when the Aura is damaged or weakened, other disease microorganisms may easily enter the body and produce harmful effects.

Consequently, a weak, depleted Aura—one that indicates reduced vitality—acts as a psychic sponge or vampire, zapping the energy of those nearby.

Without an Aura we are nonexistent; we have passed away. This Aura or Lha vitalizes the physical body. Death is our name for when our etheric body on this Earth planet stops functioning.

Different colors or dents in the Aura produce diseases. Moreover, holes in the Aura as a result of negativity, regardless of how they were imposed, create mental and physical problems. It's understood in Tibetan Tantric medicine that there are several defilements on our LHA. Defilements result from the negativity of our speech, thoughts, or deeds; the results of our past lives' or present life's karmic negativity; spirit possession; or black magic or voodoo placed on us by others, purposefully or inadvertently. The physical and mental effects incurred via these desecrations are referred to in Tibetan Tantric medicine as "wind" disease or "mind" problems. Allopathic medicine calls them psychological disorders.

Maintaining a sound equilibrium between the three components of our existence—mind, body, and spirit—is essential. One of the best methods to achieve self-healing and self-actualization is through understanding and reading the Aura—others' and our own. We can use this knowledge to protect ourselves from any external or internal negative influences, thereby keeping our temple—the Aura—spotless.

The Occidental world, or Westerners, refer to this Aura as an energy field and explain it as an esoteric body of ferromagnetic field. The Vedas explain it as energy emanating from the seven chakras. The Tantra explains that it comes from the heart seed as a result of the food that we digest, which consists of three different bodies or energies. The Westerners call this Aura an ectoplasm, and the Tantra refers to it as an LHA or energetic shadow (literally, "supreme" or "superior body." "Lama" [supreme guide] comes from the same root word). My approach is to give you an overview of all points of view: Western, Eastern (including Tantra), and new age outlooks on the Aura. In this way, you can choose that which suits you best. All opinions and systems basically agree, though, that the Aura is a reflection of us, our twin in the energy state—the real us that lives on forever.

Thirty years ago, Kirlian and now more recently Guy Coggins invented cameras that register the Aura's light energy. With such measuring devices, indicating Aura properties and characteristics, these experiments and studies helped provoke curiosity. Their work also served as reinforcement that continues to inspire additional scientific verifications, validating the Aura's existence. All this activity gave rise to newfound attention to something that the ancient clairvoyants always knew existed and were able to see with their naked "third" eye.[1]

In 1774 modern scientific research of the Aura began with the Anton Mesmer. This research continues worldwide to the present day in parapsychological research centers. Thanks to this research, skeptics with an atrophied third eye have reason to believe those with third-eye vision, or at least have their interest piqued about the Aura's existence.

Many people have heard about the Aura; books around the world have been written about the subject. In spite of all of this information, few people have an accurate idea of what the Aura really is—not to mention how to perceive it, how to interpret what we visualize, and better yet, what to do with what we know.

All books address the banal and mistaken approach of color visualization as the way to perceive and diagnose the Aura. This approach only tends to confuse and impede the learner from finding the real truth. Since all of the Aura's microcosm and macrocosm consist of vibrations, and vibrations create frequency, and frequency can be measured in megahertz, we know—as all shamans do—that color can be deceptive to teach to others because our perception of colors vary with time and evolution and from person to person. This can occur both environmental (i.e. shades of colors vary according to climate and atmospheric changes) and our own individual visual disabilities. In both cases either affecting our color perceptions and ability to see color at all. Within these chapters I offer many examples of how color can be confusing and what alternatives to color visualization are available. Controversial as you might find this concept, is also based on the fact that the human Aura is constantly changing. Therefore, color reading alone is insufficient to derive a clear and profound meaning and understanding of an Aura's condition. Auraology encourages individuals to find their own personal way to achieve Aura perception, skipping the color phase, and to *perceive* sensations.

If, however, you feel more comfortable with the color phase, multiple charts appear to help you with your diagnostic interpretations.

This book (with the assistance of the Aura goddess) serves to clarify the how-to of reading Auras as well as giving you exercises so that you can apply your newly acquired skill of Aura reading. The newfound awareness that results can give you some control on your life: more intimate understandings about it and its path, as well as about life's obstacles, so that you may grow and evolve freely. In a simple, straightforward manner, this book gives you the tools to overcome your stumbling blocks.

This fluid field of external radiation surrounds and energizes all human beings and is both material and immaterial. Contrary to popular opinion, you don't need to study for years as a Buddhist monk or Native American shaman to visualize it. Anyone and everyone who spends the time and effort to develop, practice, study, and understand their forgotten sixth sense can see Auras.

A case in point: In Italy during a meditation and an Aura reading lesson to a group of junior high students, one of these kids said to me, "I saw [visualized] myself, but it wasn't me, because I had this big widely opened eye in the middle of my forehead." It *was* him. He was envisioning his Aura with his recently reopened third eye.

Learning to read the Aura—when applied properly—can benefit our everyday lives in a simple, clear-cut, practical manner. This acquired skill can help us avoid health problems, make business decisions, improve interaction with others—even something as simple as preventing a negative or stressful encounter with someone because you have predetermined that person's mental state. All this anticipation of potential problems just by reading Auras? What a deal! Don't you agree?

This book puts you in the right direction, opens your third eye, and reawakens your sixth sense—or, who knows, maybe even your seventh sense?

What Makes This Book Different from Other Aura Books?

With a controversial look at the real facts about Aura reading, this book

- Demystifies Aura reading and its interpretation of both animate and inanimate objects, allowing each reader to believe that all are capable of reading the Aura.
- Dispels false ideas and techniques of Aura perception found in other books.
- Illuminates Aura perception, associating frequencies with sounds and color.
- Humanizes the topic with multiple anecdotes and case histories.
- Offers concise guides for body, mind, and spirit self-healing.
- Backs up theories with scientific evidence.
- Divulges simple but useful shamanic secrets to achieve self-governing of mind, body, and spirit.
- Gives several options of discernment for Aura reading, based on the author's own teaching and Aura reading experience—including, but not limited to, an excursus of several ancient cultures and philosophies. Readers can use the information to understand their own way of Aura perception and interpretation.
- Describes the spell-binding argument from the Tibetan Tantric point of view through, for example, somatic and shamanic medicine diagrams.
- Promotes a professional ethic for those who wish to help others through Aura reading.
- Explains interventions necessary to obtain a healthy psychophysical state of health through the technique of meditation and Tibetan rituals.
- Offers practical tools in a simple, straightforward manner.
- Delineates techniques for achieving newfound awareness to apply directly to your personal life.

PART 1

Aura without Color

History of the Aura, Its Properties, Its Life and Purpose

Chapter 1

What Is the Aura?

Of all the branches of occult science, one of the most interesting is the study of the Aura. Scientifically, the Aura is a subtle, magnetic emanation generated by the ether gases and other forces of the being or object[2] with which it's connected, creating frequency.

Everything in nature, all organic and inorganic matter, reflects this energy or magnetism. The fact is equally true of the lowest crystal and of living organisms of low and high consciousness.

Webster's New World Dictionary defines "aura" as "a particular atmosphere or quality that seems to surround a person or thing." All matter reflects an energy field, and even though the objective is to develop your capabilities for reading and interpreting *human* Auras, for the sake of illustration and practice we use various materials and elements.

The ether field being generated reflects the energy of the spirit of the particular individual or object. For example, a team of excavators and scribes in Gravina Puglia, Italy, at a famous ancient archaeological dig asked me to help fill in missing information gaps about some of their ruins and artifacts. This archaeological dig site, as they understood it, was more than twenty-five hundred years old—a sort of city of God, that is, a divine city where all faiths and all disciplines of people lived together and ruled together). The archaeologists have reason to believe that in the highest hills of this acreage was the legislative center of all these faiths with their respective temples. In the center was a senate house where the heads of the various religions made regulatory and legislative decisions regarding the daily conduct of the town citizens. They did not tell me all of this, of course, prior to escorting me there. They handed me some pieces of rocks and indicated to me others still imbedded in the ground and asked me to identify their purpose. The rocks contained some indistinguishable etchings. They wanted to know if the markings were just the result of years of erosion or if indeed they were some sort of calligraphic impressions of the time. Taking the stones into my hands, feeling them and using psychometrics,[3] I began to feel and hear a woman sobbing. Peering more deeply into the Aura of these rocks I saw three people: a boy about twelve years old, a woman, and a man. I sensed that they were the parents of this young man. This adolescent was a student monk. In fact, the odor of burning ritual herbs permeated the psychic environment. Within the Aura I saw the woman crying. I felt her despair because her son was no longer with them. In fact, he was cloistered in a distant monastery. I visualized him walking out to these very rocks and beginning to etch a message to his parents. In my clairvoyant opinion, they were a series of cryptic messages telling them to be happy for him because he was at peace and joyful to have found his vocation and true purpose in life.[4] These inscribed rocks bore the images that represented a series of letters back and forth between the three—the only way they could communicate, because the young man was not allowed visitors while he was studying.

My report confirmed for the scientists and their scribe that the adjacent dig was indeed what they had thought it was: a monastery. Of course, coupling this with other proof, they arrived at the conclusion that these rocks were truly to be left intact and not to be removed.

This reading also gave them some insights into the lifestyle of the time. Historical accounts indicate that the ancient religions of the Orient took children at age nine (as in the case of the present Dalai Lama) and put them into monasteries if the astrologer/ monk determined that they were an important reincarnation. Indeed, in the Aura of this rock I saw a very special child: one who was illuminated with a white light. I also sensed an incense like perfume similar to South Asian / Indian spices.

The information I supplied regarding this dig, collected through psychometrics, put together with the scientific facts gave the archaeologists the final puzzle pieces they needed. Filling in this and other information voids helped them arrive at a more concrete understanding of the era and the value of their excavations.

Of course, the ability to read an object's Aura represents a more advanced state of consciousness. Not everyone is able to achieve this level of expertise, but the point is that psychometrics is another aspect of Aura reading. Whatever another person has touched leaves a lasting energetic impression of the person's subconscious and conscious states of mind when the object was touched. If the person is deceased, the information might stop there; if the person is still alive or reincarnated, the information reception continues.

All of this energy, commonly called the *ether field*, expands in the case of most people about two to four inches around the body. There are exceptions I discuss later, and in some layers of one's Aura, the energy field might reach twenty-five feet. The Aura reflects what appear to be various shades of the same basic colors. The spectrum can range in color from white to black, indicating presence and absence of color, to pastels to deep indigo and violet.

The textures and patterns in the Aura's colors reveal much information about a person's physical, emotional, mental, and spiritual states of mind, conditions, or modes of being. An Aura is like a thumbprint; it's completely individual and expresses who you really are in your entire splendor. It indicates your past, present, and future mental states; your previous lives; your destiny; other entities that surround you; your character; and your weaknesses and strengths, whether they are physical, pathological, emotional, or psychological—*the Aura is the real you.* Your best friend. Your life's companion. It needs to be nurtured, understood, and guarded—protected and safeguarded against injury, damage, or loss of life with the same watchful and concerning eye of a sentinel responsible for the safety of a fort.

Analogies, Scientific and Other

Is there any practical and scientific proof of the existence of the human Aura? Yes, and its existence is manifest in various ways.

Let us first consider the common magnet. Around its poles, writes S. G. J. Ouseley in his book *The Science of the Aura*, is a sphere of influences known as the *magnetic field*, through which passes lines of force between one pole and the other.

You see evidence of this field when watching the influence of a magnet upon light iron filings. When these filings are placed at random on a sheet of paper, they respond to the magnet held beneath them without contact, and they follow the motions of the magnet. If the magnet polarizes these small filaments there is a remarkable affinity in their motion; they become temporarily imbued with magnetic power.

If these filings possessed intelligence and could be questioned, they would probably say that they moved because they desired to do so. The filings readily followed an irresistible impulse. They would not be conscious of the real source of the power. The more sensitive the filings, the greater the distance at which their response takes place. Consequently, the more sensitive ones would respond readily to impacts that would have no effect upon the filings of lower sensitivity. Movement converts the motion into power, and this power may be transformed into light, heat, or other forms of energy. This phenomenon is known as *induction*.

In the human organism there are forces analogous to, if not identical with, the forces of electricity and magnetism. Each human being possesses a magnetic field: the Aura. It radiates from each individual, as solar rays emanate from the sun. The human Aura partakes of the essential qualities of an individual's etheric, astral, mental, and spiritual forces. In a vital sense, every human being creates their own magnetic atmosphere, which unfailingly reveals a person's temperament, disposition, character, and health.

Practical proof of the Aura's existence comes in many forms. For example, when charged with high-potential electricity, the Aura itself becomes electrified; if a neon or argon-filled lamp is then brought within the "sphere of influence", the lamp lights up. The illumination occurs within a definite boundary, which varies around the body—but there is a definite line of demarcation. In this way one can definitely map a person's Aura. The image is much like the output of a computer-programmed pressure-point peripheral developed by a German clairvoyant, used to measure and register the human Aura for the purpose of prognosis and diagnosis.[5]

These spheres of light extend to various widths, depending on the person. This boundary could be a matter of inches in one part and possibly a number of feet in another. The lamp rays can be traced in a straight line for five or six feet.

Another interesting and recent innovation is that of Luciano Muti: the psychic sensor. This sensor uses a laser to intercept brain waves at a distance. This piece of equipment (a computer program and its decoder) makes it possible to document and measure human mental psychokinetic influences. Unlike other computerized devices used to measure the human Aura, the psychic sensor demonstrates, via a graph, the frequencies of the brain and their capabilities, as well as the subject's diseased organs.

Many idiomatic expressions attest to the Aura's presence. We hear people speak of a person's "magnetism" or someone "having a certain aura." Consider the expression used to indicate someone's power: their "sphere of influence." All these idiomatic expressions come from the concept of the Aura.

Occult scientists have known about Aura emanation for a long time, under a variety of names. It's the "magnetism" of Mesmer, the "electric fluid" of Jussieu, the "odylic flames" of Reichenback, the "exteriorized sensibility" of deRochas, the "vital rays" of Dr. Varaduc, and the "prana" from Vedic practices.

Many parapsychologists using strict laboratory controls over their methods and equipment have built on such psychic research, which covered shamans, healers, and even nonhuman elements or materials. All agree unequivocally that all bodies, animate and inanimate, emit a subtle radiation, and that we emit and are composed of vibrations. Special sensitivity is, of course, needed to detect subtle forces in nature and the Aura. Although most people in ordinary states of consciousness cannot detect an Aura, it's discernible and clearly recognized by the same individuals when they are in suitable conditions or have stimuli that permit them to perceive at their highest capacities. We all demonstrate some level of this inherent power in different degrees at varying moments of consciousness. One of the most common to all people is telepathy: for example, when you think of someone and then the phone rings, and it's the person who just came to your mind.

The human brain can be in an altered state of consciousness, a relaxed state that allows our natural capacities to function at their best. This altered state occurs when we are in the *alpha* brain-wave stage; such as that brought on by meditation and in the first few and last few minutes of dreaming (also known as the rapid eye movement [REM] state).[6] The more highly evolved perception of this state is called "clairvoyant" sight.

In ancient times there was testimony to this subtle extension of the soul. For example, the halo surrounding the head of a saint is no poetic or fictional terminology, anymore than is the invisible Aura or sphere of life radiating from a precious stone. Sometimes this Aura portrayal is not restricted to the head; it's also depicted in antique artistic renderings as surrounding the whole body with a misty glow or luminous cloud.

Another historical account is Moses coming down from the Mount with the stone tablets with the skin of his face shining such that people were unable to look at him.

I reflected the same glow more than twenty years ago during a near-death experience. Having been a crime victim I began passing into the layers of death. During that state while traveling through the light, I experienced an apparition at the end of it of the Holy Ghost and Jesus Christ. Flying above them closer to me was St. Rita, my guardian angels, St. Michael the Archangel, the Blessed Mother, and this strange figure I did identify until many years later: the Buddhist goddess Vajrayogini. She is symbolized having a skull cup in one hand, drinking from it nectars that nourish the brain and mind; in the other hand she carries a ritual spade that cuts away at negativity. This yogini represents those who work as shamans or psychologists. At that time the monks told me I should be initiated in the Vajrayogini *pooga* initiation (a Tibetan ritual dedicated to a female Buddha, Vajrayogini) and some time later taught me the Vajrayogini ceremonial dance between a male and female.

During my voyage, having experienced a profound sense of finitude, my deepest desire was to continue the journey to the deepest depth of the light. But the figure I identified to be God the Holy Ghost (the Christian symbol of spiritual and mental awakening) told me to return because I had not yet completed His work on Earth, and that I must go to Italy for Him. During this episode I felt an exhilaration, exaltation, and total peace I had never before experienced. It was quite enchanting. I wanted to continue the journey into the final depths of that tunnel—toward this luminous ray of light. Having a sense of duty to mankind and a strong reverence for God and His orders, my logical mind pulled me back. Even though I wanted to continue this voyage into the strata of death, I returned at His will and against mine. Now I work in Italy also and even resided there for over eleven years as He requested. Since I decided to commit to this calling, my life has revealed itself slowly and vividly on its own wings. The transformation is occurring in a Zen-like fashion, to the point that not only is God giving me opportunities to promulgate my prophecy and philosophies in Italy, but throughout Europe, Egypt, Canada, and the United States. Next stop? I'll ask my friend Aura.

For several weeks following my near-death experience, I continued to feel this same elation. Two to three hours after my return to consciousness, my childhood friend Stella visited me. Stella, who had never seen an Aura before, told me to her astonishment and amazement that I was completely surrounded by a luminous white light that extended at least one hundred feet outward from my physical body. She also commented that instead of demonstrating physical stress due to a violent attack, as she had anticipated seeing, I had a glow of peace and harmony; my skin was incandescent and perfectly smooth as silk, and my eyes radiated the innocence of a newborn baby.

These intense examples of luminescent white light are examples of an Aura that is lit by the infinite power of the Spirit or the Buddha inside each of us. Modern-day new agers call it a *spiritual consciousness*. As Stella experienced, these very strong Auras are easier to see and sense, which is why I use a volunteer who possesses a stronger, more illuminated Aura when I begin guiding people in Aura reading. A less intense Aura or an Aura under stress is more difficult for the beginner to perceive.

The Aura is a subtle extension of the personality, which is capable of both giving and receiving impressions. Through this medium we make conscious or unconscious contact quite apart from our physical senses. Even though many of us are *right now* not aware of our Aura, from time to time we have experienced a strange power brought about by the very force of our personality or mental state at that moment—a sort of animalistic radiation or instinct, such as when a person is "on the prowl." When their wishes come true, it's because they are unconsciously transmitting their availability. They give off a corresponding musklike odor to a receptor or interested party . . . and it happens! Two etheric bodies are sending out the message, "I'm available!" They eventually find each other. The lesson? Be careful of the messages you give out if you're not ready for the consequences.

The romantics call it *attraction* and *repulsion*. I call it an intrinsic harmony or disharmony between the Auras. This is one example of the Aura itself sensing. Another example is when a person enters a crowded room and ferrets out another person in particular. When you approach that person you find an immediate compatibility. That's the Auras at work in a karmic sense.[7] Whatever the reasons—previous lives or present life—is not under scrutiny here. The important point is that these cases reflect the Auras melding together for a particular need fulfillment.

One of the layers of the Aura is our astral body (Tibetan Tantra: Illusory Subtle Lha). Another example of the Aura at work is when clairvoyants sense the presence of a nonliving entity (spirit). Clairvoyants are sensing the ectoplasm or astral body, the etheric counterpart of the being that is envisioned. The Aura is also that astral body that flies and travels or astral projects from place to place at will, such as accounts of high gurus in levitation. These astral voyages also explain out-of-body experiences such as when I passed through the so-called tunnel of death during my near-death experience. It's not the physical body that moves; it's the Aura body. Some historians and theologians speculate that Jesus Christ didn't die on the cross, nor did his body resurrect. Instead, He projected His Lha or His ether body. In fact, some scholars say that Jesus, during those inexplicable thirty years of absence from the human record, was studying in what is now

India with some yogis and learned astral projection, or out-of-body experience.

In the same group of Italian children that I referred to earlier, almost all had the sensation of rocking during meditation in search of their Aura. An observer would have seen that no one's physical body in the room swayed. Instead the children felt their Aura's astral body beginning to leave their body. It undulated back and forth, attempting a trajectory. But because the energetic body did not yet have enough propulsive force, it left and returned, left and returned. This back-and-forth motion created the oscillation sensation.

Another case in point of astral traveling is when spirits of the previously incarnated (deceased) have not yet reached their final destination. It's their ectoplasm, the etheric counterpart of the being, that we see, not their physical body. In order to take on a physical form, these spirits suck energy from whomever they are near. They have no physical body. That form is only temporary; they arrive here and become visible via astral projection with their ectoplasm. (The Tibetans have a more profound explanation, which I give later.)

Beware of the Curve in the Road

There are various ways to explain what an Aura is and how it's formed. The color indications vary. The shapes within the various layers vary, dependent on cultural and personal mores and a person's background. I find it difficult to believe that there is only one way to interpret Auras. I don't even care that much about the explanations for the different methods, and neither should you. Look upon the various interpretations or reading guidelines only as indicators, as guideposts in the road.

Dr. Tom J. Chalko says, regarding the Aura, "Nature gave us all we need to see Auras. All that is required is knowledge on how to use your senses together with your conscious effort. If you decide not to try, you will never see the Aura. When you *see* something for yourself you no longer need to rely on believing someone else. You will know—as I do—because experience is the best teacher." Seeing Aura will only be the beginning. You will learn even more.

In the interest of instructing the novice and skeptic simply and convincingly, I offer a variety of explanations regarding different aspects of the Aura. Because the postindustrial world seems to need logical explanation, we use these for the sake of indication or guidelines only. Again, I urge you to use good judgment and not to dwell too much on rational explanations, but I am sure you will find them interesting.

I've experimented with all the methods you're about to discover. I've investigated them, taught them, and received feedback about them from my pupils. All these ideas have been processed through the trial-and-error method. The simplest thoughts for the Western mind are the best. If you digress from these recommendations, you'll risk getting too hung up on the whys and not be able to successfully achieve the dos.

Do not complicate your lives too much with explanations and examples. Begin *here and now* to experiment with Aura reading. With this in mind, skip the following chapters of this book for now, so as to not be influenced by the intellectual explanation and go directly to chapters 6 and 7 on meditating for the practical exercises on visualizing the Aura. Then come back to these chapters.

The Tantric explanations are more profound and more complicated for the Western mind, but in my opinion they are more on target than any other explanations. Whether it is the Tantric way of analysis or the modern-world mode, for many reasons I'm not interested in dwelling on any explanations, no matter how logical. One reason is that it requires much more study to profoundly comprehend the Tibetan approach, or even the other, more simplistic philosophies. Second, we are already bogged down in over intellectualizing the simple things of life; too frequently we fail to smell the roses because of analyzing their scientific characteristics. When we do the same thing with occult experiences we lose perspective of the sixth-sense aspect. Approaching the subject matter first from the intellectual point of view and then attempting to achieve an emotional experience makes it more difficult to bring our innate though unused senses back to life. Instead, we have to jump into the feeling aspect, first and foremost.

Too much emphasis on the intellectual aspects of our questions pushes us more in the direction of logic and less on perception. At that moment our experiences and perceptions become superficial and incomplete. If you continue this modus operandi with Aura reading, you will find it harder to see with your third eye. Making the transition from one brain hemisphere to another—from the rational side to the intuitive side—is often too difficult for the average bear.

Let's stop becoming victims of the adage, "We have eyes and we do not see," and move on to bring our third eye much more sharply into focus.

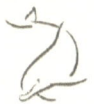

Chapter 2

Why We Need to See the Aura
The Everyday Aura

After many years of trial-and-error in instructing, I know that these techniques—combined with student willingness, readiness, and diligence—are idiot-proof, somewhat like the revolutionary computer software manual *DOS for Dummies*. Through this approach and insightful teaching, I have not lost a person yet. Everybody perceives something. Those who stick with it are able to employ these methods for such purposes as self-actualization and self-healing and to find out the real meaning of life. Achieving this state can also help a person prepare peacefully for death and the dying of others. What are some everyday applications of seeing the Aura? Some examples are as follows.

Physical and Mental Well-Being. Seeing an Aura makes possible the early diagnosis and informed prognosis of diseased areas, perceiving indications of successful healing from physical mental and emotional diseases, and discovery of past lives and karmic missions. When I or any other qualified mystic reads an Aura, we read the malfunctioning in the body long before symptoms become evident. We can see the "first residence" of disease in the outreached, profound spiritual layers of a person. By reading your own Aura in combination with color or frequency visualization, you can consciously control your Aura and actually heal yourself. These layers and colors correspond with organs that eventually become diseased if not prevented from being absorbed into the next layer or destination, which is the psychological/emotional;

the final destination is the physical whole or hollow organs, which correspond with those channels or line of currents.

Spiritual Development. Healing of the physical body is nothing compared to what seeing and reading Auras can do for our consciousness, spiritual development, and awareness of nature. Certain Aura meditations (according to Tibetan tantric philosophy and practice) build a basic level of Aura health and harmony, thereby purifying, healing, strengthening, and protecting the Aura and our chakras, and thus helping us safeguard against an otherwise polluted world and environment.

Business. Aura interpretation can be utilized to anticipate a person's mental or emotional state before having a business meeting. Depending on whether you are in the buyer's or the seller's seat, the specific advantages are many.

I remember one of the most critical meetings I had as a very young New York executive and the sexual distraction factor that my female presence often created during business meetings. Being a female executive was a strong disadvantage in many ways, since the majority of the decision makers were men. Being men, big at woman hawking, they concentrated more on my physical attributes than on my intellectual skills. So, first, on the evening before a major decision-making presentation to this corps of macho men, I visualized myself being calm and not aggravated or embarrassed by their sexual glances; second, I protected myself from any mental invasions by them and bathed my Aura in the appropriate frequencies. Before walking into the conference room, I read their individual and collective Aura. I then changed their predominant negative colors from *desire* to *rational.* This shift made them less emotionally visceral and more intellectual and levelheaded. At that point, they were predisposed to evaluate my proposal with pure logic. This always worked to my favor, because the proposals were sound.

Romance. Reading Auras can be a good tool for a more successful engagement or marriage by letting us know when our partner is ready and open to a certain discussion. When we first meet a certain person, if we see that our Auras don't mix well, that individual is perhaps not for us. Maybe the Aura will let us know that we are only supposed to be with that person for a limited period of time for certain karmic reasons. An Aura can reveal when and if the time comes to split or not to split; or when to begin to embark on a relationship with a person. Following these understandings, we can accept the outcome more readily and less traumatically, insulating us against the breakup depression blues. The clarity of the whys of being with the other person and our mutual destinies offers us easier acceptance of the events, and we live with less remorse and melancholy.

Sex Lives. Reading an Aura can help us avoid sexual conflicts with our partners. Learning about your own and your partner's Aura is one way to understand the nature of complex, intimate and sexual relationships. For instance, a person with a dominate red Aura might wonder why his purple partner doesn't seem interested much in sex and would rather be absorbed in some romantic novel than be intimate. Knowing this you would understand immediately that a person with such an Aura would rather daydream, fantasize about sex, and play with images mentally rather than actually having sex at *that* moment. A partner would begin to understand this and be able to handle the situation in a loving way and without doubting the other's sincerity. This tool is powerful, given that the majority of the love conflicts arise from doubts, suspicions, and insecurity.

Avoiding Anger and Confusion. Through Aura readings, one can begin to understand the inherent differences of other people and can then release confusion and anger when problems arise. For example, people with a predominantly dirty blue or red Aura often suffer from mental confusion and are always in conflict with themselves. These folks are often unstable and destructive, and they cannot necessarily keep tomorrow promises they make today. If you know not to count on their word, you will not be frustrated by disappointment that in the long run creates anger, anxiety, and chaos in your life, not to mention loss of time and money.

Everything in the Universe is just a vibration—every atom, every part of an atom, every electron, every elementary particle, even our thoughts and consciousness. As I previously explained, the Aura around living (conscious) objects (people, plants, etc.) changes with time, sometimes very quickly. The Aura around nonliving objects (stones, crystals, water, for example) is essentially fixed unless targeted by a human mental thought process. When we sufficiently influence the living Aura, we can also gain power over these vibrations. The first step is to begin to see them; the second step is to interpret them; and the final step is to utilize this newfound knowledge to gain control over the controllable and to understand when things should be left to rest, or as American teenagers say, "Let it go." "Get a life." In other words, we should not obsess or fixate on any particular event or occurrence. Avoiding obsession invests you with power—what the Tibetans refer to as *detachment*.

Attachment (the antonym) is one of the three ignorances[8] that cause disease and block us from completion of our missions in life, according to Tibetan medicine.

Because the etheric body is so eminently important to our existence and well-being, knowing it intimately gives us power over our mind and possibly alters our destiny, offering us day-to-day peace. Just imagine a world with less conflicts and illness, an Earth where we can choose our leaders on the basis of their Aura, a better place to live just because we all recaptured our natural ability to read and interpret the Aura!

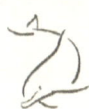

Chapter 3

How It Looks from a Tantric and Occidental Point of View

There are four facets to perceiving and interpreting the energy of the Aura. Layers are determined by vibrations. They overlap each other and are distinguished by shape, consistency and clarity of color, all within the various layers.

In the simplest terms the Aura is made up of sections of energy. There are five major (plus one dream state) Aura layers in total, according to the Tibetan Tantra; seven, according to Ayurvedic and Chinese philosophies; three, according to some new age or modern theories. Each section serves a specific purpose and relates to a particular component of a person's life. These sections of the Aura are then divided again into energy layers (vibrations), which might manifest in an illusion of color.[9] Colors can be constructive or destructive. An Aura can stimulate or depress, repel or attract, be male or female in its character, and can reflect positive or negative.

Auras more or less surround the physical body in the shape of an egg, although not a perfect oval. I call this the tent or dome. This dome has other zones within it that are less defined in shape. These abstract shapes emanate from and correspond to the various chakras. Ayurvedic culture recognizes seven chakras; Tibetan medicine uses five chakras. Within the context of the section, each layer of color displays a characteristic of the subject. The Aura also expresses itself by color tones, as well as different shapes within that basic egg-shape configuration. These three bodies, layers, or zones all overlap and superimpose each other.

CHAKRA TABLE

Impure Mind	Transformed Mind	Chakra	Elements	Petals
Black	White	**CROWN** Perception, sense of identity	Space	32
Red	Red	**THROAT** Voice, sound, taste, seat of attachment	Fire	16
Blue	Blue	**HEART** Memory, happiness, seat of anger	Water	8
Yellow	Yellow	**UMBILICAL** Body guide, responsible for embryo development, seat of pride, ambition, and greed	Earth	64
Green	Green	**SECRET** Responsible for reproduction and heredity.	Air	32

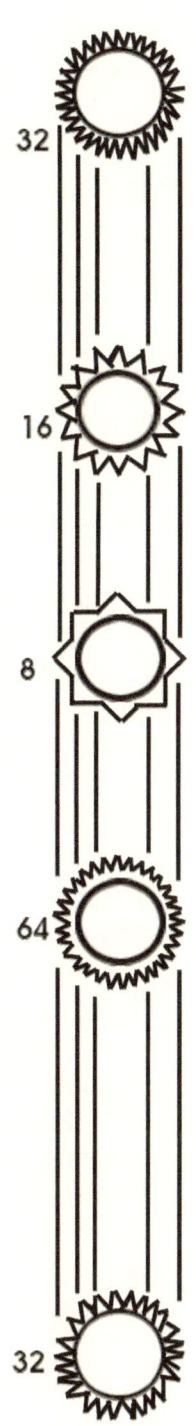

The Crown Chakra is generated by confusion. Confusion is headquartered in the brain. The results are mental defects such as fear, a closed mind and stupidity. On a physical level these provoke Phlegm energy, mucous fluids such as in the nose and brain fluids.

The causes of Heart Chakra disturbances are aversion, hatred and pride. On a physical level these provoke Bile problems. The Heart Chakra determines the ardor of a person.

The Secret Chakra is the cause of attachment and primordial instinct.

The conscience is strong sexual desire.

The Central Channel is like a "great brain" that pushes humans to enter the world. This desire on a physical plain becomes excessive Wind energy. It is this excessive desire that when misdirected can create dementia and eventually insanity.

The Occidental world offers its interpretations and corresponding explanation for each one of these layers as well as how many there are. For example, the Western idea is that the etheric body extends only a little beyond the periphery of the physical and constitutes the inner Aura; that the astral body with its egg-shaped configuration forms the second Aura; and that the mental body, with its subtler and less defined structure, forms the outer Aura.

Area and Extent according to Tibetan Philosophy

I tend to follow the Tantric explanations and less the Western viewpoints because of firsthand visual experiences, and frankly because this approach offers me a sounder comfort level. My beliefs, by the way, were in place before I studied the Tibetan point of view.

The three types of normal auric or subtle body phenomena are called the *Srog*, *Tse*, and *Lha* as well as more subtle astral bodies such as the *dream body*, the *bardo body*, and the *illusory body*. For the sake of brevity I address here the first three: the Srog, Tse, and Lha.

We have different types of physical energy. The vitality (life energy) of our gross physical body is called the Srog. An athlete, for example, has strong Srog energy. This Srog is the same thing that the Chinese refer to for sake of acupuncture treatment as the *Chi* energy. Our life span is based on a subtle energy called Tse (life span or life force) that circulates through our subtle Aura body, which radiates from the indestructible drop at the heart and is called the Lha or life essence. The Aura helps to sustain our life and consequently surrounds the very subtle mind at our heart. It forms a powerful protective shield around our body, an energetic immune system protecting us from many negative energies and diseases. At the initial stages of reopening our third eye we see the Srog, and we will gradually be able to perceive the differences between the Srog and the Lha.

The Srog is the densest type of subtle energy and can be seen extending a few centimeters out from the physical body. The Lha (Aura body) can extend many feet or meters from the body in case of powerful individuals. The Srog of a person is the vitality of one's physical body. The Tse of a person is one's life expectancy. In much of the world, a person born today is likely to live into their mid-80s, and beyond.

The most efficient areas for the average Aura reader to work on are the Srog, Tse, and Lha.[10] With this understanding alone, we can reinforce our vital energy and our health and have more positive energy to divide or pass onto others.

The Srog or physical vitality is composed of Chi. The Srog is the larger of the subtle phenomena of our body, consisting of five Chi that circulate in their respective channels. Many alternative medicine therapists use these channels for therapeutic practices, especially those based in the Orient and Mid-Orient.

Our Aura body consists of seventy-two thousand subtle channels and is like a network of seven hundred principal channels. This life span (Tse) permeates the whole body and is a vehicle that transmits the reproductive fluids (*tigle/bindu*) throughout the body from their source—the "supreme drop" (*tigle/ chenpo*), which is located in the center of our heart chakra. This supreme drop is the basis of our physical and mental health as well as our enlightenment. When the drop is activated by wisdom winds (*yeshe llung*) inside our central channel, our mind and its energies become conducive to enlightenment. When the drop is activated by the energy of our past negative deeds (the karmic winds), the mind and energy become dispersed and many mental and physical problems arise. The great tigle at the heart chakra is the size of a small pea or mustard seed and has a five-colored glow as it contains the pure essence of the five elements—earth, wind, fire, water, and space.

We can even check the strength of the Tse by examining the pulse as well as the intensity of the Aura of the life essence and checking how many breaths we normally take in a minute. This calculation tells us, for example, how much time a person has to live, or if the person's consciousness is displaced by another consciousness, such as in the case of mediums and oracles. You can actually see the other being moving within the Aura. In addition to *feeling* the entity in the pulse, you can *see* it moving up and down the medium's arm, as is also the case with negative possession. This visual proves that another Aura body has entered the person's gross body. We can also confirm these and other possessions via a fresh urine specimen.

On the other hand, the Western explanation seems to be that it's all a series of distinct layers that can extend from eighteen inches to two feet. Instead, the Tantra indicates that they overlap in a sort of three-dimensional fashion. I visualize and interpret the Aura in the same manner as the Tantra explains. Of course, strangely I saw it that way prior to my studying anything about Tibetan Tantric medicine.

The important thing for you at this point is twofold. I firmly believe that how we see and what we see and how we interpret these readings is individual and personal and only comes with practice and trial and error. For example, if we see that a person has hardening of the arteries, we need to confirm it with them. Until you've done this dozens and dozens of times you will never be sure of what you're interpreting. When you compare your impressions against the confirmation from the person whom you are reading, then and only then do you know what your third eye is telling you. After having developed a sense of security you instinctively develop your personal thumbprint for reading and interpreting—remembering, of course, that just like thumbprints, each person's Aura is unique. I've never seen a duplicated Aura. Even within the same day, one person's Aura can change from the early morning to the night. So don't be discouraged if you see the same person in the morning and in the evening and that person's Aura is different.

According to Tantra tradition and my personal experience, many other zones exist besides these three. They reflect the subtler aspects of person's emanations. In this area, a shaman can perceive a person's previous lives' Aura or LHA. From this vantage point, we can understand a person's homework or mission in this present life in relationship to that of their previous lives' experiences. Contemporary society calls this *karmic regression* or a *past lives reading*. The Tibetans call this the *subtle astral body*, the *dream body*, and the *bardo and illusory body*. We don't address previous lives' readings in this volume because it's a really advanced state of Aura reading that requires a particular vision which not everyone can attain.

Let's not get off track, though. For the beginner it's important to grasp onto something as a guideline and to learn that all of these indications are nothing more than earmarks. Choose a method and explanation with which you feel the most comfortable and eventually you will develop a sense of security about it.

With time, the ability to see an Aura becomes to our third eye what vision is to our two physical eyes. In fact, in the beginning they appear to be one and the same because we use our physical eyes in the initial stages of Aura perception. I have designed the Auraology Jeepers Peepers—titanium, dolphin-shaped monocles—to aid in this level of perception, and the monocles also help to strengthen the retina. The Jeepers Peepers stimulate the aperture of the real "light" and "light perception" that comes from the third eye.

Aura Layers according to the Modern World

Tibetan explanations pertaining to the number of the Aura's strata and sublayers are infinite. In fact, it's too infinite and advanced for a novice or just those with only the sixth-sense perception. Most of these layers can commonly be seen and fully comprehended only by shamans.

The modern explanation, much abbreviated by comparison, holds that the Aura is made up of seven main Auras, extending up to four feet from the body. These Auras all occupy the same space at the same time, each Aura extending out farther than the previous Aura. All Auras are interconnected and rely on the others for normal functioning. This aspect is somewhat similar to that of the Tantra explanation.

The seven main zones of the Aura are as follows:

1. The *etheric Aura* extends about two inches out from the physical body. This Aura is associated with the health of the physical body. In this Aura you feel all sensations, pain, and pleasure. Whenever there is pain the flow of energy in that area of the etheric Aura is erratic.
2. The *emotional Aura* extends about two to four inches from the physical body and appears as rainbow-colored clouds.

This zone is associated with feelings. Problems in this Aura eventually lead to problems in the first and third Auras.

3. The *mental Aura* extends about four to eight inches from the physical body. Within this Aura are our thoughts and mental processes. Thought forms are also found within this Aura.

4. The *astral Aura* extends eight to twelve inches from the physical body and serves as the bridge between the physical world and the spiritual world.

5. The *etheric template Aura* extends twelve to twenty-four inches from the physical body. The etheric Aura has an empty groove into which the etheric template fits. The etheric template Aura holds the etheric Aura in place. It's the template for the etheric dimension.

6. The *celestial Aura* extends about twenty-four inches from the physical body. This is the level of feelings within the Spirit World.

7. The *ketheric template Aura* extends about thirty-six to forty-eight inches from the physical body. This Aura takes on the form of an egg that surrounds and protects everything within it.

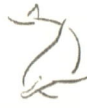

Chapter 4

How the Aura Develops, according to Tibetan Medical Science

According to Tibetan medical science, the auric light body is a natural result of the transformation of food essence into the seven bodily constituents of food essence (*chile*), blood, muscle tissue, fat, bone, bone marrow, and regenerative fluid. When we eat, our body transforms the essence of our food into seven stages to produce seven physical constituents, the subtlest of which is the auric body. These seven transformations are as follows:

1. The food that we eat is digested and absorbed into the blood. This food essence circulates in the blood, and its pure essence transforms into blood. The waste returns to the stomach as mucus.
2. The pure essence of our blood transforms into flesh, and the waste goes to the liver and gall bladder as bilirubin. (Bilirubin is a reddish-yellow, lead-filled bile pigment. It's essentially a waste product, formed when red blood cells die and hemoglobin breaks down.)
3. The pure essence of our flesh transforms into fat, and the waste is expelled from the eyes, ears, nose, mouth, and pores of the skin in the form of tears, wax, mucus, and sweat.
4. The pure essence of fat transforms into bone, and the waste becomes the oiliness of the face, skin, and feces.
5. The pure essence of bone transforms into bone marrow, and the waste forms the nails and the hair.

6. The pure essence of bone marrow transforms into the white and red *bodhichittas* (semen, egg, and menstrual blood), and the waste product lubricates the inner organs, urine, and feces.

7. The pure essence of the semen and menstruation transform into the body light (Aura) and the waste product into our hormones. In women, breast milk is a by-product of the white bodhichitta.

The Aura is considered to be the purified essence of semen and ovum; the impure part of this essential male and female energy is the semen and the menstrual blood with which we are familiar. The main seat of our body light is inside our heart chakra and is called the *indestructible drop* (or supreme drop). This is the seat of our deepest level of consciousness. The light that radiates out from it, beyond the limits of the physical body, is called the Lha, the Aura.

On the gross level, the white bodhichittas produce the embryo's bone tissue and from the bone marrow arises both the semen and breast milk. The red bodhichittas produce the blood, flesh, and skin.

On the subtle level, the red and white drops support the life essence (Lha), which sustains the physical body.

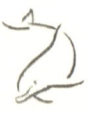

Chapter 5

Seeing the Aura

Practice, observation, and testing our observations against feedback from the subject are the tools that develop the power of Aura sight. Faith and open-mindedness are the sine qua nons. Without these essential ingredients, success is impossible. When you are motivated to try, and when that motivation is coupled with positive results, the satisfaction and sense of accomplishment reinforce increased success with each attempt.

The second rule is to trust your gut instincts and never second-guess your first impression. Just go with the flow. I realize that we are talking about working through a dimension that is not visible, and therefore skeptics find this concept difficult to swallow. But it's a reality. Yes, everyone can do it. In order to open up this new awareness, all you need is the *knowledge*, seasoned with lots of *faith*, *open-mindedness*, and *plodding repetition*. Then comes a series of graduated glimpses, and eventually you culminate in complete Aura visualization.

When first embarking on Aura envisioning, most people can be placed into one of three categories. One group consists of completely open-minded people who probably already remember some sort of paranormal occurrence but had no one to guide them through it. Such is the case of almost all children, who invariably have some episodes of these types of visions but were suppressed and scoffed at by those around them and consequently shut down. I know personally such an example: a twelve-year-old Italian boy, my meditation and yoga student. From his first day of guided meditation, yoga, and Aura reading of his fellow students, when asked for volunteers to describe what they were seeing, he was always the first, raising his hand immediately. I knew this young man was filled with untapped and undirected power. He not only saw the first layers but many others as well, in addition to various elements and formations inside the Aura. He was always accurate. The boy told me later that he always saw his mother's Aura, but was afraid to tell anyone for fear of recrimination. As a result he was able only to see his mother's Aura, not recognizing it for what it was and fearing going beyond that. After having been encouraged in meditation class, feeling a sense of accomplishment, and comprehending his power, he came to see all Auras without effort. Then the problem became the reverse. He needed help controlling when he saw and when to shut it down. Before gaining his new consciousness, this child manifested and posed a particular behavioral problem—lack of concentration—to the obvious consternation of all of his teachers. He had special attributes and was not understood, having no one to encourage or enlighten him as to his sensations and their responsibilities. Feeling more at home with himself, he calmed down and started to pay more attention in class and to apply his intellectual capabilities with enthusiasm.

The second group of people who embark on Aura visioning are open-minded and ready to learn. They likely heard about Auras but did not realize that everyone could see them.

The third and final group at first are the most difficult: the close-minded skeptics. In my experience, though, once they've acquired the capacity to see and read Auras, the former skeptics often become the biggest and best disciples.

To all categories, I say, rest assured that Auras exist. Begin with this idea and belief system regardless of scientific verification or lack of it. This outlook or acceptance is what brings you rapidly to glimpses of realizing your goal. Then your reward become firsthand verification. Once you see for yourself, you believe. Until then, you're a sort of Doubting Thomas: if you don't touch it, you can't believe it.

So let's go feel it, together, step-by-step, through meditation.

Also understand that the time line to visualization varies from person to person. Your success rate relates to you and you only, not what anyone else experiences. Before proceeding to Aura reading, read and heed the warning below and post it near your meditation area.

Warning! Management advises against ever comparing your success and results against those of others. Your experience and growth rate are unique and so are those of others.

Remember: Seeing the Aura is natural to all of us. Now relax, and let's begin to stretch those lazy muscles slowly and persistently.

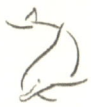

Chapter 6

Meditation and What It Has to Do with Aura Reading

Many people today are curious to see and feel the Aura. If you really want to see it, you need to create certain situations and conditions: the most critical ingredients to success seem to be a very open, relaxed mind and a predisposition toward your first practice subjects. As a neophyte, you may find your perceptions of someone blocked if you feel strongly against or indifferent toward them. If you become fixated on some aspect of their body or mind, either you will not see the Aura or it will disappear. Auras are like gnomes or soap bubbles; they appear, but if you try to grasp them, they disappear.

As your chakras are purified and developed, a meditative state of subtle vision becomes easier. For an even-keeled, easily facilitated beginning, it's important first to develop this form of sight through meditation. With the help of meditation you can first see your own Aura and eventually the Aura of others with much less effort. The first task is to arrive at understanding your own Aura, its significance and interpretations. With this applied practice you eventually start to see yourself as a spiritual individual who has occasional human lapses or experiences, and you stop seeing yourself as a human who has occasional spiritual lapses. With time you come to understand in the very depths of your heart that the most important subtleties of life are the ones that should take precedence in your walk toward Truth. Your daily life becomes less propelled by materialism. You begin to comprehend how an excessive regard for worldly concerns brings only heartache and frustration. Then, in turn, the highest value of your life becomes your spiritual well-being. You no longer believe that your physical well-being is directly connected to economic well-being, but rather to internal peace. With this in balance, you have found the Truth that helps you place a higher order to your life.

Financial success is the by-product of proper motivation. When financial gain is provoked in this manner, you find yourself wanting more and more to discover why you were placed on this Earth. What is your homework here? How, via profession or career or vocation, must you manifest this wonderful gift of existence of being alive? When you achieve this understanding, then and only then does money fly into your hands. *Lakshme*, the Hindu word for "money," which also means "energy," is the energy exchange for our giving out spiritual satisfaction. Thus, the significance of the word "money" is not material but abstract. Consequently, when we acquire a take-it-or-leave-it attitude about money—when it becomes less important, not *the* driving force or raison d'être of our existence—we automatically detach ourselves from its importance. When this driving force is exchanged for a fire and force for spiritual growth, then and only then do the dollars fall out of the clouds and land where we want them to, and keep coming. After all, even money is a vibration—a vibration which represents an exchange that dispels avarice.

They say that money is the root of all evil. But when the root of this money tree is self-fulfillment, it no longer has roots of evil, but proper motivation. Indeed such motivation can serve us well. Above all, we change our perspective about money; we no longer risk losing it and retain it. Psychologists say that an excessive desire for money results from our insecurity and narcissism, manifesting itself as a fear of being without money. That fear in itself is a result of our fear of death or impermanence. When we acquire an attitude of spirituality and detachment, our interior vision becomes clearer because we no longer make it our sole, driving goal. We shed our fears, and money is no longer the cart that draws the horse but the horse that carries us to our bliss.

At this level of realization, Aura reading also becomes clearer and more profound. Control of our sixth sense is never be taken away from us as long as our objective and motivation remain pure. Just take your time and don't expect too much too soon. Excuse the banality, but Rome was not built in a day.

Developing Aura vision through meditation, as indicated previously, is the quickest and most direct method. Any other system for self-reading won't work very well, because it's more difficult to read ourselves with our physical eyes. For example, many people suggest gazing into a mirror. I don't suggest it for the reason just mentioned: we would be relying on our physical sight and risk not seeing the Aura or projecting that which we wish to see in ourselves. But we *can* utilize our opened physical eyes to stimulate our third eye when we begin to practice reading others. However, even when reading others, we must first meditate.

In the following chapters I give you quick and simple meditation and visualization exercises. Read and practice the first one before beginning to practice the others; perhaps you will achieve what you want from the first. If the first exercise does work for you, go on, one by one, to the others.

Some students say that seeing Auras in candlelight or at dusk is easy, but probably their minds are more relaxed in that situation. Seeing Auras in broad daylight is entirely possible, irrespective of the coloring of people's clothes.[11] Later on, the Aura appears more easily and is less obscure and more opaque. Seeing it becomes a natural, normal event in your life.

Once you can see Auras, you can read people's emotional states, health, and life energies directly, even if they put on an emotional mask. Literally, when you see Auras, you are seeing people and yourself in a whole new light (excuse the pun).

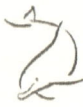

Chapter 7

Meditation, Self-Realization, and Self-Healing Techniques Made Easy

Meditation techniques are the subject of this chapter, specifically those techniques designed to help you with seeing and interpreting your own Aura and other people's Auras, as well as with self-healing and self-actualization.

Many exercises and suggestions exist for the aspiring Aura reader, both objective and intuitive. One exercise in particular, however, I personally dissuade you from trying: use of an anatomical Eye Pattern Schematic Chart. I'm categorically against this approach, based on overuse of our left-brain hemisphere (the thinking side).[12] This schematic chart might be effective for some people, but in most cases it only reinforces old habits of intellectualizing and using our physical eye. Instead, I say to go for the golden ring right away, using the sixth sense immediately. For those of you who totally refuse this method or want some assistance in getting started, however, Auraology has formulated some fashion-fun titanium eyewear as an aid in Aura sight development while stimulating the right brain.

If you want to attain Aura visualization, swiftly and with less confusion and anguish, engage the direct method. Use exercises that employ right-brain stimulation. Do these straightforward, no-nonsense techniques, which combine meditation and Aura perceiving. Proceed in the follow manner:

1. Meditate, perceiving your own Aura; 20 minutes of exercise a day for one week. (You will find the instructions for Self Aura Perception in Chapter 8).
2. Jot down notes on your experiences while meditating.
3. Meditate, then open your physical eyes and observe your volunteer subjects' Auras.
4. Jot down notes on what you were able to visualize.

Why We Meditate

Mass confusion still exists in the Western environment about what meditation is. Is it something that everyone can achieve? When do we know if we are there? These questions are the most often asked. Part of the reason for the misunderstanding is that many of the techniques engaged are too complicated for the Western mind. Everything I recommend is necessarily uncomplicated and practical. First, we should understand why we mediate.

Because thought is energy and the property of the Aura is energy, the images you visualize are manifested or created by the ethereal or (spiritual) plane. Meditation is used to provide added focus and positive energy to the manifestation of these images. This is an intuitive method of reading Auras.

Portrait conceptualized meditation can help you protect yourself, as well as prepare your surroundings for positive and enlightened Aura readings through mental projection.

In general, meditation improves our concentration and helps us to become universally centered, happy, calm, and creative. It opens up our subconscious mind at will. It puts us in an altered state of consciousness; our mind is under our control, as opposed to hypnosis, in which another person controls our voyage. During the altered state of consciousness while meditating, we are completely aware of what is happening and we self-direct. While under hypnosis, we consciously are not aware of what we see or hear or feel. Not only is another person controlling our journey, we are in a deeper frequency that does not allow us necessarily to remember or to be mindful of the occurrence or visions.

The brain-wave frequency during meditation is called an *Alpha* state. To understand this more fully, we should explain more about how the subconscious mind functions, as opposed to the way the conscious mind works.

The conscious mind is the seat of organized brain activity. It controls sense perception and expression. When you are consciously focused on an activity, your brain emits electrical waves. The *Beta* brain-wave pattern is a term commonly used to describe the wave pattern emitted in consciously directed activities.[13] It is the state most commonly experienced when we are awake. Because you over identify with your intellectual faculties, you either ignore the subtle perceptions of life or miss them entirely. They just whiz past you unnoticed.

An Alpha brain-wave pattern occurs during relaxed states, and in Alpha patterns, the brain wave registers a frequency of about 10 cycles per second. The more relaxed you become, the slower the brain-wave pattern and consequently you are more sensitive. Only about 10 percent of your body and brain activity is consciously controlled. Through meditation and Aura healing, you can improve the DNA and RNA functioning of your cells and cerebral endocrine system. Scientific documentation, through the aid of electronic equipment, during these altered states indicates that the stimulation of cerebral neurons during meditation puts endorphin and serotonin into circulation, which is responsible in the human brain for mental concentration, lessening of tension and stress, profound dreaming, and anxiety relief. If you reawaken the more subtle perceptions that register within you, you are wired to acquire serenity, happiness, mental concentration, and with reconditioning, easier access to your subconscious mind.

Concentration allows us to acquire knowledge as well as the ability to penetrate deeply into the underlying meaning of both the energetic and intellectual information and facts being presented. To be able to perceive the Aura we must be relaxed, calm, and open-minded. When we couple meditation and concentration with Aura reading and Aura healing, there is no limit to the depth or how far we can go into our personal understanding.

After having attained this ability, linked with the mastery of the Aura, we become endowed with a corresponding ability to condense bodies of facts and information into a structural framework, revealing a deeper or more synthesized meaning than what is immediately apparent to the superficial or distracted observer. The concentrated consciousness then acquires the potential for more rapid spiritual growth because of its ability to see relevance and connection between events, thus comprehending the causes behind the nonapparent causes and effects that continuously boggle our scattered consciousness. More people with such consciousness can help clarify our socially confused mental state.

Once having successfully explored Aura interpretation, we can then embark on learning Aura healing. Holding the two together we are equipped with an arm and an armature to reveal everything about ourselves; our past, present, and future lives; our mission or homework in this lifetime; and karma from past and present lives' regressions. We can protect ourselves from further harm or repetition of negative actions. We can even find out who we were previously. In the case of the highest yogi and lama, they can even choose and prophesy their future reincarnation.[14]

Without some form of meditation, the inability to concentrate grows worse. The uncontrolled circulation of thoughts and impressions in the mind or the narrow-minded picking apart and holding on to a false reality—in part or whole—or any distortion of fact limits if not eliminates the ability to provide effective analysis.

Case History

An Italian male, thirty-nine years old, was adversely affected both physically and mentally. He lived in certain negative patterns from childhood. He was reared without love and affection as a result of the consequences of a chronic alcoholic mother. One of his continuous traumatic flashbacks was his memory of finding his mother lying on the floor in the kitchen and picking her up. Absent her ability to display affection because of her constant state of inebriation and disorientation, and absent the presence of any other adult figure willing to acknowledge her problem or to give *him* love, this child lived in constant fear and confusion, incapable of understanding his life. Worse, he felt responsible for her actions. He was subconsciously certain that *he* could make his mother feel better. Having not felt better, he perceived failure.

Only as an adult did he come to understand that his mother suffered from alcoholism, because she recuperated through Alcoholics Anonymous and divulged this to the family. But her recovery came too late for him to be in control of his self-doubts and fears. The patterns were already established. We know from many previous studies of children of alcoholics how debilitating the situation can be, especially without professional guidance to help the family through the situation. Often, in some way, shape, or form, the alcoholic's offspring repeats a similar pattern and is burdened by an extreme degree of insecurity. Studies also indicate that if a child between the ages of birth and six years old does not receive the required emotional attention, many psychological deficiencies occur, not to mention the prenatal physical damages from the effects of the alcohol. These scars are quite difficult to mitigate. Some of the effects are mental confusion, lack of control of the individual's life, and complete and total mayhem that can impact any one of life's many aspects. At the all-important developmental age when children need affection, love, and acknowledgment from their parents, our subject was giving the care to his mother. It was a noble deed of love transmission on his part, without a doubt, but harmful for the possibility of his having a healthy psyche. In his young mind, he felt rejected and unloved and, later on, responsible and guilty for his mother's state of inebriation: *If only I could have saved her. She is doing this because I am a bad boy. Because I cannot save her I am to blame. Why does she drink?* Because of his insecurity and confusion, he was unable to concentrate as a child, and as a student he became known to his teachers as a troublemaker and discipline problem. All he was seeking was the attention missing from his alcoholic mother, not to mention his father, who wanted to ignore all of this by staying away from the house as much as possible and burying himself in his business life.

As an adult our subject began to understand his negative behavior pattern. *I must be the sacrificial lamb for everybody. It's my fault. It's the only way I can get attention! To help the suffering. I don't merit love.* To this day he cannot understand why his mother drank. Therefore he will move on to unconsciously make up for what he could not do before: save her.

Consequently, he surrounds himself with relationships that put him in the position of being a professional lifeguard at home and at work. Not only that; he is copying his father's pattern of staying away from home—working as much as possible and not confronting or admitting the problems he has at home with his companion, a woman who suffers from sexual codependency and engages in outside sexual relationships that psychologists suspect to be a form of nymphomania. Dysfunctional families commonly repeat the same relationship as their parents in one way or another, picking up and covering up for those who figuratively fell down and abused them.

The mother is okay now, but our subject is not. He continues to let things just happen, leaving himself prey for those who want to kick him. This vicious cycle of emotional codependency and abuse is familiar to him. After all, that's what he knows and what he's used to. That's his learned response. In fact, when confronted with a love relationship that treats him as he deserves to be treated—lovingly, supportively, in a sexually gratifying manner—he unconsciously runs, timidly. In fact, he goes so far as to question why his love has never been requited. Unfortunately, this man still carries with him the psychic damages of not having had affirmation or affection during early childhood.

As indicated earlier, chaos and mental confusion lead to life mismanagement. He has no control of his life, but he thinks he does have control, although he is always reactive and conditioned by others (even though he often rebels). He is never proactive. He refuses to really believe and see himself in that framework of behavior patterns. The same way that his mother's illness dominated his life, he accepts his companion's domination. His will, determination, and desires depend upon this dominant figure.

Why? This man is mentally confused, the same mental confusion that his mother knew when she was pregnant with him and then after his birth.

During pregnancy the baby's body is being constructed of the material the maternal organism brings it, a fact known from a remote time period. The emotional and mental states of the mother are transmitted to the baby via hormonal energy, according to the most recent psychological research placed into evidence. Tibetan physicians say that the interior or internal state of the mother affects the material of a baby's organs during their formation. Thus lies the rationale for psychological, psychosomatic, and physical illnesses.

On a physical level, our subject suffers from bouts of chronic diarrhea, intestinal blockages, indigestion, stomach enlargement, and occasional migraine headaches, among other symptoms. He has a very bad relationship with food in that he disdains mealtimes and is even allergic to many types of foods. He has had all his teeth extracted, starting first with the lower gums. The explanation comes from both medicine and psychiatry: one who suffers from allergies, asthma, or lower mouth problems can be documented to have had difficulties with the maternal role model; he associates the kitchen floor with her chronic seizures. The kitchen is where we ingest and digest food. All of this explanation contributes to what Tibetan medicine calls a *bile imbalance*, which disturbs the digestive tract. Such imbalance is otherwise directly related on a spiritual level to the remote cause of mental confusion.

This weakness adversely affected the reproduction of the brain enzymes, the neurons responsible for will and determination, thus freezing his ability to make a decision. He does not fight back by getting out. When one suffers from this impaired orientation, as in the case of this particularly gifted and intelligent person, the mind vacillates between what the subconscious mind is saying and what the intellectual or conscious mind is saying. The dialogue becomes muddled and indistinguishable. Therefore, such people become immobile and static and let the currents of life and other people make their decisions.

In these situations, a conflict arises between what the soul is telling them and what the excessive ego (also a cause and result according to Tibetan medicine) does not allow him to reveal. Such people cannot remain centered or focused on any one fact for a long enough period of time to be able to truly evaluate and understand the problem at hand. Since their fundamental style of living needs revision, that task seems overwhelming and bleak. Consequently, this thirty-nine-year-old has difficulty clarifying or admitting much about his life, even when confronted with proof about it and connecting it logically and rationally with his actions. Even according to traditional medicine, this is a common symptom of addictive personalities and their offspring: distorted logic. During this phase of suffering, these subjects lack the grit to grow, move forward, and live happily.

Meditation can help people sort out each and every one of these sufferings of sentient beings, reinforce the enzymes required to gain will and determination, and then gather the ability to do something about one's problems and live serenely.

The uncontrolled circulation of thoughts and impressions in the mind or a narrow-minded picking apart of events causes this mind "boggling," as does holding on to false realities of certain aspects of these impressions.

The imagination or image-making faculty as in the above case history continuously conditions our hopes and fears. It conditions our attitudes, which in turn affects our environment and what happens to us, thus conditioning our emotions and images again, in a never-ending, sometimes vicious cycle. For example, in this case it's guilt and lack of courage that leaves our subject prey to repeating his childhood patterns. He tries to compensate for what he could not achieve for his mother: saving her. The cycle continues, as he repeated the same trauma with a drug-addicted and now deceased cousin. To the present he voices his frustration at not having been able to save him. This insurmountable behavior creates gaps between his inner life and his outer environment. Since he has sought little or no opportunity to ever look at, confront, and sort out these gaps, he will not emerge from this perplexing way of living. His childhood restlessness that was once manifested as a lack of interest in intellectual pursuit (schoolwork) and a little bit of the bad guy toned down as an adult. Now, instead, he throws all his energies into work and accumulating material items. He is becoming an adult locked into these patterns as the social mode of existence and he rebels, but his rebellion is misdirected, manifesting itself by occasional explosions of anger and sometimes violence.

Referring to the Intrinsic Nature Table, you can see the cycle of desire leading to dissatisfaction leading to anger.

TABLE: INTRINSIC NATURE OF A HUMAN BEING

The Three Relationships between the Organic Channels and the Chakra Mental Defects
(contamination and excessive energy)

The mind is the root of all illness. According to Tibetan Medicine the less we are attached (dependent) the more happiness we incur.

Bile, Wind and Phlegm are universal energies. We, the microcosm, are part of the Universe, the macrocosm. We are constantly connected to this macrocosm. That is why our mind and body is subject to changes that are impacted by the Universe and vice versa. *Bile* and *Phlegm* (positive and negative) correspond to the yin and yang and are connected to the material aspects and the energy. *Wind* is neutral.

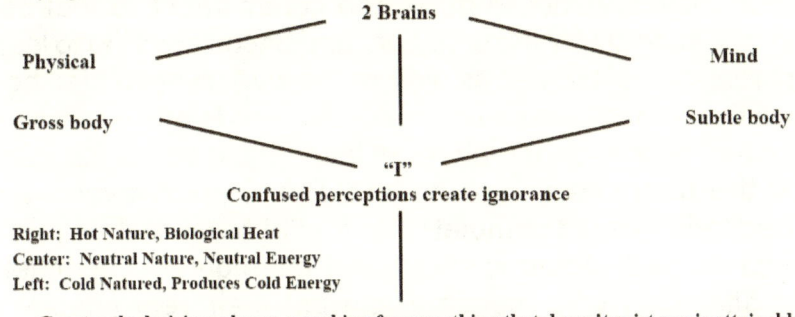

2 Brains

Physical — **Mind**

Gross body — **Subtle body**

"I"

Confused perceptions create ignorance

Right: Hot Nature, Biological Heat
Center: Neutral Nature, Neutral Energy
Left: Cold Natured, Produces Cold Energy

Constantly desiring, always searching for something that doesn't exist nor is attainable

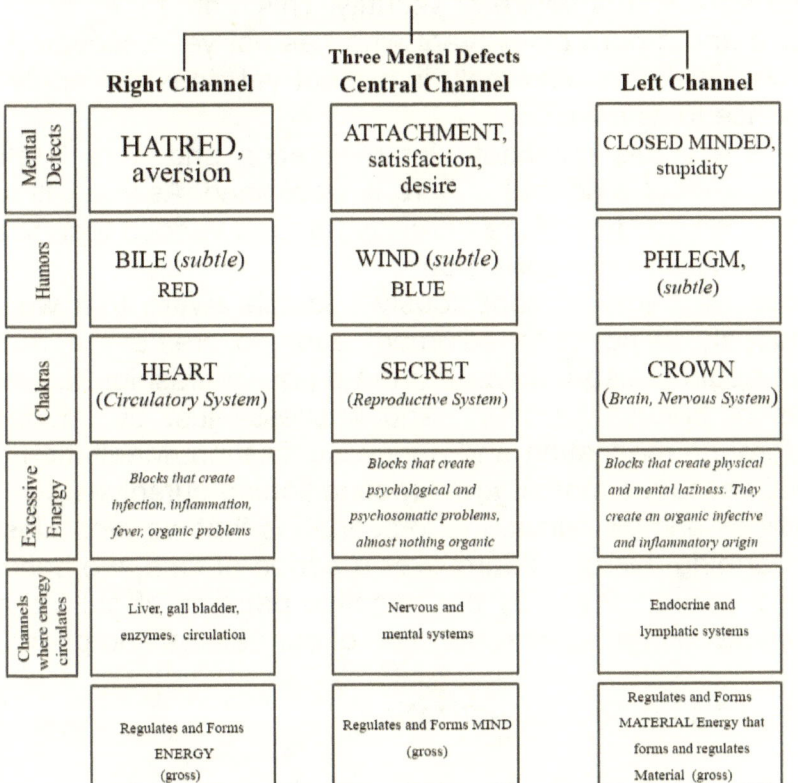

Three Mental Defects

	Right Channel	Central Channel	Left Channel
Mental Defects	HATRED, aversion	ATTACHMENT, satisfaction, desire	CLOSED MINDED, stupidity
Humors	BILE (*subtle*) RED	WIND (*subtle*) BLUE	PHLEGM, (*subtle*)
Chakras	HEART (*Circulatory System*)	SECRET (*Reproductive System*)	CROWN (*Brain, Nervous System*)
Excessive Energy	*Blocks that create infection, inflammation, fever, organic problems*	*Blocks that create psychological and psychosomatic problems, almost nothing organic*	*Blocks that create physical and mental laziness. They create an organic infective and inflammatory origin*
Channels where energy circulates	Liver, gall bladder, enzymes, circulation	Nervous and mental systems	Endocrine and lymphatic systems
	Regulates and Forms ENERGY (gross)	Regulates and Forms MIND (gross)	Regulates and Forms MATERIAL Energy that forms and regulates Material (gross)

More importantly, his karma is not being worked out. Either his life will grow increasingly worse until he tries to stop this process, or in his next life he will carry forward the same tendencies, which might manifest in an even graver manner. Oriental philosophies understand that until we work out a particular karma it keeps getting worse and worse until we deal with it properly and move on with our development.

If our subject wants to make the commitment to feel better, make the time to clarify the situation, and become willing to learn to accept real love of himself as well as the love given to him, he can achieve this through structured meditation and yoga exercise—on the spiritual as well as the physical level. We discuss the spiritual level in the Tantra section of the text. The physical level is simply that meditation would stimulate his frontal brain and help him to reinforce his will, determination, and courage. He or others in similar situations who meditate can put their very special gifts into evidence with a sense of security. This man, for example, is sensitive and a born clairvoyant who has not yet discovered his clairvoyance. He is extremely intelligent yet does not apply his intelligence to its fullest.

He is a viable candidate for meditation and Aura healing, because without a doubt his Aura is weakened. As you will read later, we can build our Aura intensity through various techniques that help with karmic regression.

Once we begin to consciously become aware that we are continuously using distorted imagination to create our reality, we can begin to use the same art in a positive fashion to create images of beauty, harmony, and success—just by imagining them through meditation and auric visualization. Meditation and spiritual passages that suggest reconditioning ourselves change our images and visualizations to scenarios that we most desire. By performing this procedure over a period of time, we become less and less enslaved by the negative patterns of our life and more involved in positive realization of our desires and peace.

Self-Healing for Self-Actualization

These activities of the mind are the norm, do not yield high-level thinking, and certainly don't require genius. The discursive thinker or casual observer does not have the ability or the power to develop his or her mind into an instrument that directly perceives the real behind the apparent until the necessary faculty of concentration is developed. Concentrating one's mental energy pierces the veil into deeper levels of meaning, to which all great scientists and philosophers testify. Of course, going from the idea or vision or ideal to the reality is quite a step. To manifest the above objectives and goals requires steadiness of purpose, knowledge of method, and proactivity. Self-healing is acquiring the capability to use our energy for ourselves in order to obtain liberation or self-realization, and then to use this actualization to heal and help others achieve the same goals. Self-actualization or self-realization is a gradual, unfolding process, and we must be prepared to exercise the needed patience along with the needed perseverance to achieve it.

Because the subconscious mind controls an estimated 90 percent of body and brain function, an open and relaxed mind is of utmost importance. Put it all together and you'll see that meditation offers the best method for high concentration and mental clarity. Which is why it should be used before every session of auric sight development, self-healing, and self-actualization. Do so until meditating and seeing the Aura become an automatic conditioned reflex. Many advanced practitioners can walk in the street in the middle of traffic and still be meditating and visualizing Auras without major effort.

Meditation Preparations

Physical Surroundings (Selecting an Environment)

Choose a spot in your house or garden to use habitually for each exercise. The most ideal spot is a private corner or room in your own house, as it's surrounded with your energy. As you know, the longer and more intimate the contact you have with a place, the greater familiarity there is. This familiarity becomes a comfort zone because your traces of energy are there, kind of like a male feline that sprays its environment, carving out its territory. Proof of the pudding is that your bedroom feels different from your brother's bedroom or your parents' room that might be in the same house. Second, your house or your corner of the house is under your control as far as privacy is concerned. Think of it as the architectural version of Linus's blanket.

The actual place isn't that important—unless it's a place that really distracts or irritates you—as long as you are comfortable, feel secure, and can control the energy flow in the room. It's important, though, that the blanket is clean and spanking new.

This does not mean necessarily that you must elaborately re-design your space. It is best to pepper these tips with personal needs but to be certain that it is an orderly clean space

Items Needed

Speaking of Linus's blanket, choose a rug or floor cover that is yours and yours only. Wear loose-fitting clothing, preferably white or light colored, never black. No shoes. Never mix energies and swap blankets—metaphorically—with another person when performing energy practices such as meditation and Aura reading. The reason is simple: Based on the energy exchange principle, during meditation you leave your energy behind on your prayer shawls and blankets. They are energized with a particular frequency of energy—called "essence"—of meditation and praying. *Your* soul state is projected, leaving traces on whatever material you use. Each time you use an article for meditation or readings, that item becomes even more magnetized and you'll find it easier to achieve and hold a meditative state of mind when in its presence.

The same is true when you use an article that belongs to someone else. Do not use others' hand-me-down clothing. In fact, there is even a prescription that Tibetan physicians give when someone suffers from wind or *llung* disease (in Tibetan medicine) and Aura detachment—not to use clothing or personal items of any type that belong to or were worn by another. It adversely affects your Aura.

The most ideal yoga/meditation carpet is one of natural fiber, such as a lamb's wool "yoga" carpet, that blocks the negative ions of the atmosphere. This blanket should be at least the height and width of your body, if possible. Otherwise, any natural material is fine. Don't spend a lot of money on it. If you visit Eastern countries you'll find that they don't even know about commercialized yoga carpets or pillows, but they manage to meditate just fine.

Lighting and Environmental Effects

There are many suggested methods for preparing a room for a reading. Until you find what works best for you, I suggest natural indoor light, but a few well-placed, soft light fixtures can do just as well. Judge which to use depending on the comfort level you require for concentration. Dwell in a place where you will not be disturbed for at least an hour, a place without distractions. I do not recommend the outdoors for the beginning meditator, because finding an isolated place where you hear only the sounds of nature is most difficult. But if you find one, by all means frequent that environment. Avoid a room that is bombarded by electrical devices, such as computers, televisions, or stereos. If it's not possible, at least make sure that they are disconnected from the electrical outlets. Turn off cell phones and disconnect the battery.

Dim the environment of natural light by lowering the blinds, but allow the light to come through in a limited fashion. Many people use a lit candle. Many even concoct a triangular-shaped tube in any natural substance to sit under because it attracts positive energy by its form, just like the pyramids.

Native Americans use smudge sticks to replace negative energies with positive forces from the Great Spirit. Tibetan shamans use revolving prayer wheels and twenty-five-ingredient natural herbal powders to chase away the evil spirits. The ancient Celts used a knot mandala or a nail to capture and block evil spirits. Many people arrange selected crystals in specific patterns throughout a room to ward off any unwanted energies. Some people employ a combination of all of these. Simply choose the ones that suit your personal taste. In all cases, prepare the room before you begin.

Tape Recorder

Keep a tape or digital recorder handy for recording your self-reading perceptions. Then replay the recording later and take notes on what you saw and where. Make sure this recording device is operating only on batteries. Then later compare these notes with your feelings from those of the successive session, and so on. Indicate in your notes any accuracies and conflicts. List whatever comes to mind, no matter how bizarre it might seem. After a few days or a week has passed, review the notes and see if anything you saw has come to pass or is beginning to make more sense.

For example, if you thought you saw a faint green light around your chest but you have no physical illness in that area, go back a week later and review your notes. You may discover that the green energy was warning of the chest cold you have now.

Music

When teaching I always use a particular tape very difficult to find in the West, since it was purchased in Dharamsala. It's a recording of Tibetan monks playing singing bowls. The singing bowls have the various vibrations that heal the various chakras of our etheric body and the five elements of our physical body. In the absence of such a recording, choose a nature-sounds recording, such as the roar of the ocean.

You can even go to the beach and record the sounds yourself, including the chirping of the seagulls. Not only does it cost nothing (if you live near a beach) but it's yours personally, and the memory of the surroundings when you listen and relisten to the music will be lasting and help you to concentrate and mellow out quicker. Of course, many soothing meditation-type recordings are on the market, and if you choose to buy one of these, fine. But I highly recommend eventually recording your own. By all means, in the meantime use an appropriate music recording. Otherwise you run the risk of having greater difficulty in meditating because of distraction from outside noises and mind racing.

Body Position

Use the lotus yoga position, or the closest you can get to it (see illustration).

LOTUS YOGA POSITION

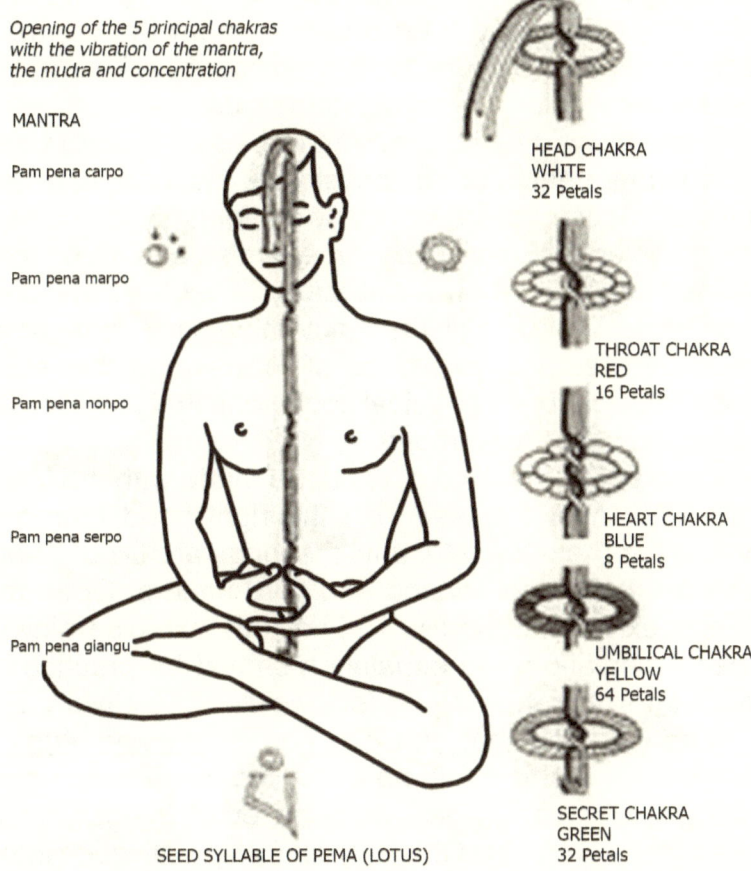

*Opening of the 5 principal chakras
with the vibration of the mantra,
the mudra and concentration*

MANTRA

Pam pena carpo

Pam pena marpo

Pam pena nonpo

Pam pena serpo

Pam pena giangu

SEED SYLLABLE OF PEMA (LOTUS)

HEAD CHAKRA
WHITE
32 Petals

THROAT CHAKRA
RED
16 Petals

HEART CHAKRA
BLUE
8 Petals

UMBILICAL CHAKRA
YELLOW
64 Petals

SECRET CHAKRA
GREEN
32 Petals

The reason for maintaining this position is threefold, but not absolutely necessary for Westerners to follow. If we find it uncomfortable or if we have some physical impediments, we can rely on the supine position. The three reasons for the lotus position are

1. Reducing the possibility of falling asleep
2. Offering proper and sufficient energy flow
3. Sitting physically in the form of a triangle—the infinite spiritual shape

Deep Breathing

The simplest form of breathing is inhaling and exhaling from the diaphragm and then breathing from the depths of the stomach. Inhale to the count of 10, then count backward, exhaling completely, slowly, for five complete rounds.

If you prefer, you can do a more cleansing type of breathing, which Tibetans teach to all physicians as part of their daily meditation practice before receiving patients. This meditation is typically coupled with a purification exercise and helps to relieve suppressed emotions but in this case I'll explain the breathing part only. The Vedics call the Anulom Vilom Pranayama. It is the safest of breathing exercises of Pranayama that should be moderate enough for all physical conditions that is instructed fully on you tube by Swami Ramdev.

Beginning of this exercise has to be made with the left nostril. Hold the right nostril closed with the right hand thumb. Inhale slowly through the left nostril until the lungs are filled. Then close the left nostril with the second and third fingers. Open the right nostril and exhale through it. Repeat this exercise slowly. This practice of inhalation and exhalation should be practiced slowly for about three minutes. I suggest viewing the Swami Ramdev video demonstration that you can find on www.youtube.com. I find, however, that this might be a little too much to coordinate for the novice, particularly when we have other things on which to concentrate. I recommend this only for Aura purification exercises, which we discuss later.

The Meditation Exercise

The lotus position is considered the first yoga position and the position of completeness. Based on the concept that we are composed of five elements—space, crown chakra; wind, our secret chakra or reproductive chakra; fire, our navel chakra; earth, our heart chakra; and water, our throat chakra. Each of these is represented by a color: space, a white circle, wind, a green bowl; fire, a red triangle; earth, a yellow square; and water, a blue circle. (See the Lotus Yoga Position chart on page 67.) This illustration helps us understand the perfection of the lotus position. Within our physical body the elements are reflected. Our heels are half circles and the shape of the wind mandala. When we sit cross-legged, our crossed legs resemble the shape of a half circle. Our groin is a triangular shape, which is why the fire mandala is located there. The abdomen is a square shape, symbolic of the earth mandala; the neck is kind of circular shape, which represents the water mandala. Our skull contains a sphere of space, where our brain sits, like the circular shape of the space mandala.

When I refer later on to cleansing methods, these types of visual meditation exercises will prove useful. But for now you need not bother with them. Put all this aside and just concentrate on the music and the following simplified practice.

> Visually divide your body into parts.
> Your head and throat.
> Your shoulders and your chest.
> Your arms and your hands.
> Your stomach to your navel.
> Your groin area and hips.
> Your thighs to your knees.
> Your lower legs, from your knees to your ankles,
> Your feet and toes.

Now you are in a sweet, quiet room, listening to your selected music, sitting in a lotus position on your very own carpet that is blocking negative ions. You are ready to perform the simplest of breathing exercises. You are inhaling, slowly, and exhaling, slowly, for five rounds each.

Now you start to give your body parts a nice trip. Visualize each and every one of them floating and relaxed above you.

You repeat, visualize, and concentrate, watching your head and neck floating way above you. Relax, relax, and visualize. Then say, "My head and neck are floating above me and are relaxed." Then, repeat, *relax* and *concentrate*.

Keep repeating the same type of instructions to each and every one of the above body parts in the above order. When finished with that part, just stay there, floating and relaxed and concentrating for another ten minutes. Then bring yourself back in the following manner:

Bring each group of the same parts of your body back, one group at a time, in reverse, starting with your toes and feet, then going to your head. Slowly open your eyes and stretch.

This whole process takes about twenty minutes. Do this for seven days, taking notes afterward on your experiences, before you try working on the Aura of others.

Before comparing these (Some of you might already be seeing colors intuitively prior to reading this book but not quite know if they are or what it means.) to the interpretation charts, do the following: If you are good at drawing, make a sketch of what you envisioned and the colors that you saw. Otherwise, record your perceptions just by writing a detailed description. Alternatively, draw or sculpt your impressions. In the group of Italian kids whom I taught, one young man hesitated when I asked the students to create a visual arts expression of their meditation. He looked at me hesitantly. I realized he felt uncomfortable with the design arts. I asked him what he could do, and he said, "I play a musical instrument, the flute." I suggested that he compose an original musical work demonstrating his feelings. He did so, the first time he produced an original musical composition. He was quite happy and thrilled to do so. His music teachers even lauded his accomplishment because it was the first musical composition by a student in his junior high school. He felt really inspired by the meditation and was doubly pleased because he was acknowledged for his musical talents.

Frequently, people start to see their own Aura from the first day. If you do, move on to the color charts and look for the health indications that might reflect your situation. For example, if you know that you have circulatory problems, look to see if you saw that color indicated in one chart or another. If you don't find the pathology or impression you are looking for, chances are that these charts will not work for you because you see different colors to indicate different things. In this case, you'll have to gradually develop your own color charts. You'll only know what's accurate for you through lots of trial-and-error testing both on yourself and others. Always solicit the feedback you'll need to discern what colors are yours.

Meditation to Prepare Yourself before Your Subject Arrives

I particularly suggest the following for reading another's Aura:
Close your eyes and take in three deep breaths through your nose. As you do, imagine the positive white light of the Universe entering your lungs and energizing your physical body. As you exhale through your mouth, imagine a gray smoke that carries with it any negativity, stress, and anxiety as they exit your body. Say to yourself: *I release all stress and negative emotions to the Universe, where they can be dissipated and no longer do harm to anyone.* As you take in your final breath, imagine a higher energy filling your lungs with a large ball of pure, protective white light.

As you return to normal breathing, imagine the white ball of light beginning to grow as it mixes with your own energy. As the ball becomes larger, the positive light pushes through your organs, tissue, and muscles—forcing any leftover stress out of your body—and is dispersed into the Universe where it will be purified. Imagine the energy pushing up through your chest, neck, and head. Then see the energy pushing downward, through your stomach, hips, legs, and feet.

When you have imagined the light fully encompassing your entire body, push the light farther out in front of you to open a doorway through your Aura. Imagine a giant pair of pure white hands opening your Aura and pushing it aside like a curtain. Ask your conscious mind to help you keep the doorway open until the reading has been completed.

Sit for approximately ten to fifteen minutes and allow a higher light to energize your body and prepare you for the reading. When you are ready to end your preparation, thank God and your inner self for their assistance.

When you're ready, open your eyes and make any final preparations for your reading.

Tips for Reading the Auras of Others

The most important step to reading another's Aura is not to let your own energy get in the way of your sight. Your energy field can act as a filter and cloud the view of your subject. Depression, anger, or any draining emotion can also cloud your vision. To combat these problems, be sure you are fully energized and emotionally upbeat when conducting a reading. This mental outlook strengthens your well-being and prepares your physical body for the energy it expends during the reading. I recommend to not do these experiments if you have a cold or flu. The reading may rob your body of valuable energy that it needs to combat illness. Having said that, the same is even truer regarding severe illnesses. Don't practice healing or Aura reading for others when you are weakened. To eliminate the filter effect of your own Aura, take a few minutes before your volunteer subject arrives to perform a brief visualizing mediation. This action temporarily moves your Aura out of the way and provides you with the clear path needed to see the subject's Aura.

You want to remove a much smaller amount of the filter if you are self-reading. You don't want the filter in front of your eyes to distort the energy around your body. At the same time, you don't want to move too much of your energy out of the way either. Doing so clears your Aura, and then you'll see nothing of value—much like erasing a videotape before you've watched the movie.

Remember to protect yourself from your volunteer subject's energy output. Energy is free-flowing, potentially affecting anyone or anything in its path. So as not to absorb others' emotions or problems, learn how to protect yourself from these external energies. This knowledge is extremely important when reading others, because you risk taking on their emotions, which is almost like being infected with a disease. Other people's energies interfere with the reading, not to mention the rest of your day.

I cannot emphasize enough the critical importance of self-protection during energy exercises and activities. I have seen and heard of too many instances of the unprotected going astrally astray or surrounded by negative forces that cause nervous or physical disorders or negative possessions.

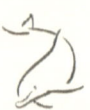

Chapter 8

Techniques for Reading Our Own Aura

Here we go. This method is the simplest and least convoluted for reading your own Aura. Of course, you should meditate first. Once you've mastered this technique, you can even use it to visualize former lifetimes.

But first, *your* Aura. You've probably already visualized your own Aura in meditation and didn't even know it. The possibility of seeing your Aura while meditating might seem strange to you, but have faith. For sake of clarity, I offer an overview of some possible scenarios for seeing your own Aura.

To provoke remembering what you saw in your mind's eye, ask your intuition the following questions:

What is the energy of your Aura?
What is the primary color of your Aura?
What other colors are there, and where are they most strongly located?
What do these colors or visions reflect on a physical, emotional, mental, and spiritual level?

Here are some of the possibilities of what you may have seen:

Multicolored balls
Blue night that you thought was black.
Only one color.
Multicolored blotches or strips.
Black and white blotches.

All of these experiences were visual possibilities during the first phases of Aura visualization.

Some if not all of you probably felt as though you were rocking. In reality you were not rocking, but your Aura or Lha was moving away or astral projecting, giving you the oscillating sensation.

What are some other possibilities?

Some of you may have had only certain physical or emotional impressions, and some might even be convinced that they have seen nothing. But if you think you saw something or even felt something inside the pit of your stomach, then rethink it through. You perhaps saw something that you were not aware of at first. You might have just ignored it as meaningless and insignificant. Still not convinced? Even if you did not yet see colors, those feelings and impressions should be noted as well. All information you gather about your experiences and responses is useful for self-healing and karmic regression.

The more open-minded might have seen actual nature scenes such as fields, deserts, mountains, and so forth.

Some of you might have heard sounds other than recorded background music. Your Aura is communicating with you. Consider this story: Once with a group of meditators I was using an old portable tape recorder to play my singing bowls tape. The tape recorder badly needed oiling; it was making a disturbing noise while playing the tape. One of the more difficult meditators shouted with glee, "I heard something! I heard this strange beating noise all during the meditation." Then he asked, "What was it?" Several of the other students shouted with laughter, "It's the tape recorder that needs to be oiled!" The poor guy was demoralized. He thought he was finally getting it. So don't try too hard. You might tend to place too much emphasis on getting it and you might not *get it* because you are overstressing and pressuring yourself with the requirement to succeed.

You might have felt a tingling or pinging sensation in some part of your body—for example, a numbness in your feet, like your foot going to sleep. This is an example of your Aura leaving your body. Don't fret about this sensation because that ping in the pit of your stomach might be your way of getting responses. This is the beginning of transporting you into an altered state of consciousness. The pinging is probably your Aura giving you a nudge. A six-year-old boy I know can only see his Aura when he first twists his nose with his fingers.

Perhaps you did not hear a thing but received information by means of a thought process. This also is your Aura speaking to you. By the way, your etheric body (the mind, by Tantra standards) can communicate with a very fine vocabulary through the use of thought transmission and reception (telekinesis). Furthermore, since your etheric body has a voice and does not get much chance to use it, it's tickled pink to have someone with whom to communicate.

As you learn to work with the etheric body, you come to understand that she has a personality. Sometimes shy, sometimes warm and friendly and eager to shout out, she even has a memory. When you repeatedly visit, she remembers you. You should make the first move, though. Say "Hi" when you enter; "How are you? I'm coming to visit you today, okay?"

Upon exiting, ask her questions about yourself that you want to know. Then say, "Good-bye, and thanks for the info."

Try making friends by developing your communications skills with your etheric body. She loves to chat and eventually gives you information you didn't even request.

These, too, are auric experiences. Whatever or wherever you are, Aura brought you there, mixing with other Aura vibrations in the process.

Whatever variations of the above you experienced, realize that you are already on your way to success.

The two methods of Aura reading are intuitive and objective sighting. You can develop this capacity in a two-step phase of reading: first intuitive sight and then objective sighting. The instructions in the following chapter are exclusively written for helping you develop the third eye only. However, you can develop a certain Aura sight using your physical eyes. Auraology has designed and developed Aura-vision fashion wear accompanied by an instruction book that aids intuitive and objective visioning.

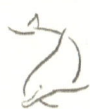

Chapter 9

Reading Others via Intuitive Sight

After having done the note taking and meditating process for a solid two weeks and experienced seeing your own Aura consistently or when you feel ready, move on to visualizing the Auras of others.

Use the same room, but now with full natural light. It's advisable to do your first experiments in full light. In succeeding experiments, divide between full light and semi-light. Use your judgment to indicate when concentration and practice have produced in you a sort of induced passivity. Then and only then may experiments be done in semi-darkness.

Remember, any extreme type of lighting is not advisable—neither bright lights nor total darkness. A soft natural or artificial light from the hallway or window is okay as well.

I mentioned earlier that your first subjects should be high-energy persons, which actually means that they have a vast, deep Aura. They are the easiest for you to visualize. You should also feel in harmony with them before starting the reading.

Now that you are adequately adept at meditation preparation, I suggest it's time to start reading others. The best time for these first experiments is in the daylight.

1. You, the reader, after having meditated, can gaze at the sky (not the sun) for half a minute. If it's after sundown, gaze at the electric light for the same length of time.
2. Close your eyes, sit down, relax, and try to become as passive as possible.

3. Concentrate mentally on the idea of the Aura. Be careful to avoid making an effort of will.
4. Place your selected subject against a white wall, about twelve to eighteen inches away from it. The person should be in a standing position, arms along his or her sides, and feet firmly placed on the ground. (I did not mention having a white wall in the section on setting up your private space because that sometimes is difficult to have and the beginning exercises are for practice—when you have a subject then it is advisable to have a blank wall to place them against, preferably white).
5. Fix your physical eyes beyond and around the person's head and shoulders. Concentrate on what you see around the person.

Gaze calmly at the subject and note the formation of any mist, lights, or rays in any region of the person's body.

Do not be dissuaded easily if you are unable to see anything. Patience and regular practice is as necessary in developing auric sight as any other form of psychic development. Colors in the Aura are not always seen objectively, but they may be felt or sensed. I maintain that our mind's eye has prejudiced the reader based on previously read and promoted concepts of color reading. The reality is that there are many ways in which we individually perceive the Aura. It could be a thought process, a ping in the stomach, or a sensation. Regardless if these sensations contain color, we still successfully perceive the Aura. Continue to read about this technique, and if you have no success at seeing or sensing colors, try this exercise independently of the meditation and the actual subject reading. People who do not perceive colors are often candidates for more strongly tapping into clearer interpretations.

The skull seems to be the main field for manifestation of the Aura. People who are above average in mental power and alertness have a much broader and more clearly defined auric base around the head than others who are less intellectual. For this reason, I recommend that you gaze on these areas of the person in your first exercises. Eventually you see or feel colors, or experience other sensations, around other parts of the body.

In fact, strong-willed people can control the energy and colors of their Aura. I proved this by changing the color of my Aura while I was hooked up in Italy to an inventor's newly invented Aura reading machine. Knowing what colors and intensity I had, I altered my Aura. In effect I was testing the machine's validity. Since our Aura changes every millisecond, that also suggests the unreliability of these mechanisms. The time delay from electronic impulse to final stage of registration within the computer program cannot keep up with the rapidity with which our Aura changes. (At least I have yet to see one yet that can.

Be careful not to choose a subject who is strong-willed and adept at changing his or her Aura at will and who might fool you and consequently discourage you. You will be confused about what you are seeing and not be able to get the proper feedback for the interpretation experiments.

For many people the first visualization is seeing a narrow, fine gray/black (transparent) circular line or band around the head and shoulders of the person, which is actually between the body and the Aura, somewhat like the halo that appears on the holy cards of saints. Another early visualization often involves the interior of this circular line, which seems to be a bluish-gray sort of misty image. Still others see that, and a very clear gray/white. These are common beginning stages for people who just don't automatically leap into seeing a full Aura layer.

If you are having difficulty at sensing or feeling something, you might not be sufficiently relaxed and consequently remain close-minded. Or you may have predetermined to see colors when it's not necessary to perceive color, but rather to *perceive*. If you still want to hang in there, I recommend a few additional exercises that will prove to you that this "energy" really exists.

Color Visualization Exercises

If you are finding color awareness difficult and insist that this is *your way*, try the following exercise under the conscious control of the mind. During the exercise, visualize the seven major color rays.

1. Place slips of brightly colored paper each in different envelopes.
2. Sit in an easy chair or recline on a couch or bed in a comfortable position.
3. Devote a few minutes to deep breathing, to bring about a state of relaxation.
4. Breathe deeply and slowly until it's impossible to inhale any more air.
5. With your chin placed on your chest and your eyes closed, hold the breath and bear the full lung pressure down on the pit of your stomach for a few seconds. After that, exhale gradually until the lungs are entirely emptied of air.
6. Make a mental picture of a globe of light that is constantly changing color. First red, then orange, yellow, green, blue, indigo, and violet.
7. After a few minutes of color concentration, hold one of the envelopes in your hand or against the middle of your forehead and try to visualize the color within.

Keep doing this exercise until you are satisfied with the results.

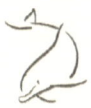

Chapter 10

Alternative Auric Sighting Exercises

At this point we should have remaining only the skeptics who are direct descendants of St. Thomas. If you identify with this description, let's move on to some easier exercises that might stimulate bridging the left and right hemispheres of your brain, allowing you to more easily make the transition.

Nature is the most admirable and beautiful love affair that we have available to us. It trains the powers of observation, leading human beings to feeling an ownership in its overwhelming loveliness. People acquire a love for plants, animals, birds, and insects, helping remove the fear of jealousy and prejudice in human relations.

Based on this premise, instead of people let's practice a little on the plant and animal kingdom. Let's go outside.

Exercise 1: See Auras around trees and plants.

You can do this one with the Auraology Jeepers Peepers Fashion Eyewear, too.

1. Look at the top of a tree with the sky as a background.
2. Look a little past the tips of the limbs or leaves of the tree/plant.
3. Let your eyes go a little out of focus and just relax.

You should see an almost glowing, cloudlike image that moves in and out from the tree/plant.

Exercise 2: See a bird's Aura.

1. Wait for a bird to land on a tree limb.
2. Stare or gaze at the bird, letting your eyes go a little out of focus. Don't strain your eyes or try too hard. You may not be able to see the Aura on the first try.

A circle surrounds each bird, and it usually has a transparent purplish color, almost cloudlike. The Aura moves with the bird, in and away from the body. Eventually, you'll perceive the Auras of an entire flock of birds in flight overhead.

Still another choice for the die-hard skeptics, if you're still having no luck . . .

Exercise 3. See your Aura coming off your fingertips.

Again, sit in a room that's not too bright. Stand in a doorway with the hallway in total darkness. The room you are in should be lit. Stand with your hands toward the hallway and your back toward the lighted room.

1. Take your two hands and make the tips of your fingers of both hands touch each other.
2. Place your hands (with fingertips touching) about eight to ten inches away from your face.
3. Gaze directly at your fingertips while moving your hands slowly away from each other (about six inches apart) as if in slow motion. You should see a whitish band between your fingertips that almost looks like a rubber band.
4. Move your fingertips back to their original position (touching) and slowly move them back and forth, touching and moving the fingertips (hands) away from each other about six inches.

Exercise 4: Test your auric radiation sight—to be done alone.

When you go to bed at night, take an ordinary iron magnet with you. Put out the light, making the room as dark as possible, and get into bed. Relax for a minute or two, making your mind as passive as possible. Then hold the magnet under the bedclothes and gaze steadily upon it. You might, of course, lift the bedclothes, but the magnet itself should be invisible to you. You can tell by touch where it is. After a few moments you should be able to see a faint, pale light hovering around the poles of the magnet. The light will vary in intensity according to the degree of auric clairvoyance you possess. You may see just a misty patch of light or clearly defined rays. If either phenomenon occurs via this process, you should be encouraged further to believe in auric existence and have the shove you need to open up your mind. If you fail the first or second time, don't give up. Keep testing yourself for at least a week.

Still another option for those skeptics who did not see Auras of human subjects: If you have not seen the Aura of others, try the following exercise in a group setting. You might benefit from the input and feedback that results from the collective energy that a group transmits.

Exercise 5: See Auras in a group.

Place the fingertips of both hands together for upward of a minute and then slowly draw them apart. Auric radiation can be seen issuing from the tips of the fingers and uniting hands. Lay a matte black cloth on a table. Relax and now try to see the Aura. By the way, you can create an atmosphere with music or group singing or chanting.

1. Lay your hands palms downward over the cloth.
2. Point your fingers toward a person opposite you. The etheric rays should be seen reaching across and uniting.
3. Look around you at the other pairs of sitters. Around many hands a dark line may be seen intervening between the fingers and the Aura surrounding them. The outer edge of the Aura emits rays of varying color and intensity. The hands of the more vital and sensitive people appear to radiate sunlight while others remain gray. When Auras cannot be made to blend, phenomena do not occur. If you

see little or nothing, keep changing partners until you find the right combination.

If several sensitives are among the experimenters, the Auras from all hands blend in the center like a luminous cloud composed of rapidly moving auric particles.

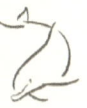

Chapter 11

Color Aspects and the Life/Death Cycle

One thing we all agree on among the various philosophies of Aura disciplines is that the Aura is the sum total of one's thought forces and emotions—the etheric, astral, mental, and spiritual life of the individual. We shall now see how the Aura expresses itself in terms of color vibrations. The basis of the study and interpretation of the Aura is the fact that thoughts and feelings collect around the physical frame in what could appear in the form of fine, vibratory waves or rays of color. This light forms a dome, tent, or protective layer that separates us from death. When the Aura is consumed or separated from our physical body, our duplicate, twin, or mirror reflection dissipates or never returns to the body and we die.

This dissipation can occur through natural life/death-cycle means (what the Tibetan Tantra calls "She" or the "Mara of Death" [see the Reincarnation Cycle illustration and the Tangha of Magic Labdron]); or it can happen unexpectedly through trauma-induced separation that speeds up the separation time; or it can happen through means of black magic or spirit Aura stealing. The concept is the same no matter how it happens. We begin to die slowly from the millisecond when we are born, according to the Tibetan medicine theory as well as the *Book of the Dead*. Death by natural or extranatural causes is always due to the depletion of our Aura by one means or another.

The Reincarnation Cycle

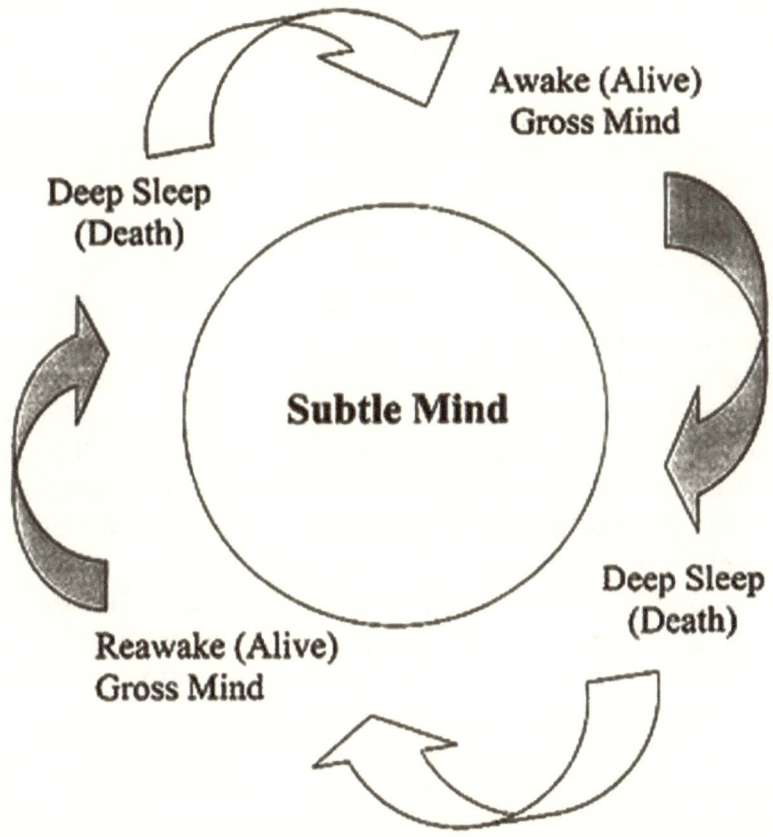

The other point on which all disciplines agree is that the Aura is a fine wisp of color. Some are denser than the others. This predominant color depends on our dominant chakra energy, emotions, and state of health. The predominant color is what a newcomer usually sees first.

The Tantra teaches that the Aura becomes more intensely colored when a person experiences good health; positive energy, thoughts, words, deeds, and emotions; and healthy spirituality. The Aura becomes less intense in color under opposite circumstances. Our Aura contracts as well.

Last but not least, the disciplines all agree that our Auras consist of multiple colors.

Now let's take a look at how the Aura experts explain the visions they see as translated into color vibrations. The basis of this collection of thoughts and feelings through our food essence becomes visible to the third eye as vibratory waves or can give the illusion of a color of light. Actually, quantum physicists refer to color as a vibration as well. Each color possesses a symbolic frequency entirely its own. The world of Nature is a symphony of color expressing emanations of various light rays, whether the delicate hues of dawn, the vivid tints of the sunset, the magnificence of the rainbow, or the intensity of the midday sun in summer. Remember, we talk about a vibration that *can* appear to be in color, but in reality it's a frequency. That is how I sense the Aura, to be able to distinguish through its seventy-two thousand layers sufficiently for diagnosis and healing. Why? Because that is the ancient wisdom reality. Most sense color when reading Auras. That's okay for the average nonshaman. It's also okay if you never gain the color instinct, as color can fool you. For example, when you look at the ocean is it really blue? Is the sky really blue, or is it a reflection of the gases and environment around it?

Some occult science teaches that the Central Sun emanates great vibratory rays or wavelengths of light termed the seven major vibratory rays from which spring the seven basic types of human mentalities and temperaments.

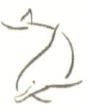

Chapter 12

The Sound and the Vibratory Nature of Man

The history of sound and vibration as associated with the human mind and body dates back to ancient Chinese medicine.

Contemporary practitioners have been endorsing color visioning and the interpretation of diagnostics and Aura perception for so long that readers still do not know that there are many other methods for visualizing our spiritual and physical body.

Changing mind-sets can be a tough job. Since my mission is to place into your hands all of the bona fide ways to read your Aura for self-realization and healing, I am willing to risk being burned at the proverbial stake for proposing that you try to reach the heights of the shaman healers. If you have never visualized a colored aura or auras at all, keep an open mind and ignore the color thing for just a moment if you can.

This book gives case histories about reading Auras and methods through which one might perceive the Aura. They range from thought processes to actual graphic visualizations. The more musical aspect is the least known and accepted by either the scientific world or the occultists.

With the help of many contemporary analysts of sacred sound, my style of working and understandings are now supported by their technical research on the subject. Although much controversy remains within the scientific community, research parallels many of my own personal experiences. As an intuitive child prodigy, I could not perceive the colors of the Earth plane on which I was born in this lifetime. I remembered in my mind's eye colors and tones that were not here. Many years of quandary and reflection revealed to me that I brought with me from previous lives not only the recognition that nature's colors used to be different from those in this century but also my recollections of feeling frequency and sounds relative to Aura perception.

Learning Aura perception by sensing frequencies and gradually associating them with a particular pathology and illness is the most accurate method of energetic diagnostics. Each individual reflects her or his own momentary color as well as one's own mode of perception. Through many years of auric self-healing, no two practitioners were alike in their diagnostic color interpretation unless they had read the same book.

The heart of every esoteric musical philosophy is that the entire universe is governed by an original sound. Sound is a form of energy resulting from vibrations.

The association of sound and color has a long history in Chinese traditional medicine. With sound we form letters, with letters we form syllables, with syllables we create words, and with words we create our daily life. Science recognizes that everything in this universe is vibration. As far as association between a determined sound and a determined color is concerned we find a divergence of opinion within these charts. Each chart was constructed by intuitive individuals' personal experiences and research, much like those that I illustrate regarding color and color interpretation—again confirming that our experiences and readings are each individual and uncertain. These charts, however, conclusively support my mode of teaching. I offer guidelines for these teachings, and I also provide individual tutoring to help you establish your way of discerning this mysterious aspect of self-healing.

The band of frequency of a piano ranges from 27½ Hz to 4,186 Hz. Within this band are established specific frequencies, for example, the notes, A, B, C, D, E, F, and G. Among the two octaves one would expect a corresponding reciprocal but it's not so. The scheme of each chart is an attempt to synthesize the relationship between colors and notes and is defined differently by different sources."

Source 1: Ancient China

Name	Note	Color	Element	Direction	Season
Kung	C	yellow	earth	center	late summer
Shang	D	white	metal	west	autumn
Kyo	E	blue	wood	east	spring
Chi	G	red	fire	south	summer
Yu	A	black	water	north	winter

Source 2: Bali

Name	Scale Grade	Color	Divinity	Direction
Ding	1	Red, blue, black, white, yellow	Shiva	center
Dong	2	White	Iswara	east
Deng	3	yellow	Mahadewa	west
Dung	4	red	Brahman	south
Dang	5	black	Vishnu	north

Source 3: India

Name	Scale Grade	Color[a]	Color[b]
Sa	1	lotus	red
Re (Ri)	2	green or orange	pale green or red
Ga	3	gold	orange and cream
Ma	4	jasmine	pale red
Pa	5	dark	red and yellow
Dha	6	yellow	yellow
Ni	7	all colors	dark

[a] Alain Danielou, *North Indian Music* (New York: Praeger, 1968).
[b] Shahinda, *Indian Music* (Delhi, 1923).

Source 4: Alexander Scriabin, Russian composer, d. 1915

Note	Color
C	red
C#	violet
D	yellow
D#	reflections of steel
E	pearl blue
F	dark red
G	reddish-orange
G#	purple
A	reflections of steel
A#	light blue

Source 5: Dyhani Ywahoo conference (Venerable Ywahoo is 27th generation lineage holder, Chief of the Green Mountain Band of the Cherokee Nation, and revered Tibetan Buddhist teacher)

Scale/Grade	Color	Corresponding organ
A	green	eyes
C	red	heart, ears
D	yellow	flesh
E	metallic white	skin, mouth, intestines
G	blue black	bones, anus

Source 6: Roland Hunt, Self Analysis Through Color—Steven Halprin, Inner Peace Music

Scale Grade	Color	Frequency
C	red	261.2
D	orange	292.1
E	yellow	329.5
F	green	349.2
G	blue	392.0
A	indigo	440.0
B	violet	493.0

Source 7. Some Color Keys

Scale Grade	Color (a)	Color(b)
C major	white	red
D major	yellow	yellow
F	green	red
F#	gray-green	brilliant blue
A	pinkish	green

B minor: "The black key," Beethoven.
E minor: "For the Young Girl Dressed in White with a Pink Bow on Her Chest," Schubert.

The following listing summarizes the color relationships. The numbers reflect the sources numbered above.

Note	Color
C	red (7), purple, green, yellow, lotus
C#	red, turquoise, green, violet
D	orange (6), yellow (3), blue, white, green, blue-green
D#	yellow, indigo, blue, reflections of steel
E	yellow (5), metallic white, reddish cream, violet, blue, gold, indigo
F	blue (2), green (4), ultraviolet, violet, dark red
F#	violet (2), infrared, brilliant blue
G	green, blue (4), blue black, black and white, red (2), reddish orange, white, jasmine
A	indigo (4), green (2), amethyst, orange, blue, red, black
A#	orange (4), yellow, reddish orange, reflections of steel
B	violet (4), purple, sky blue, lemon-yellow, light blue, yellow

When we see light, in reality, we perceive all frequencies together. The frequency of the spectrum is approximately 16 to 17,000 Hz. Randall McClellan, music professor and sound researcher, connected these frequencies with the various notes, mathematically resulting in the following chart.

Frequency	Color	Frequency under 40 Octaves		Differences	Note
430(x 10(12degree)	red	391.3	G	392	0.7
460 "	"	418.6	G#	415	3.6
490 "	reddish orange, orange	445.9	A	440	5.9
520 "	reddish orange, yellow	473.2	A#	466	7.2
550 "	lemon-yellow	500.5	B	494	6.5
580 "	lemon-yellow, green	527.8	C	524	3.8
610 "	turquoise	555.1	C#	555	0.1
640 "	blue	582.3	D	588	5.7
680 "	indigo	618.7	D#	623	4.3
720 "	dark violet	655.5	E	669	13.9
760 "	darker violet	691.5	F	700	8.5
800 "	ultraviolet	727.9	F	742	14.1

McClellan also informs us of the various studies between the relationship of color and sound, and the multiple sources and resources that point to this concept such as Roland Hunt's *Fragrant and Radiant Healing Symphony*, published in English in 1937 with an explicative subtitle: "The investigation of the marvelous correlation of the virtue of color healing, sound and perfume. The idea formulated by the author, is fascinatingly indescribable, that which in the 19th Century was considered bizarre and non scientific, above all, those which refers to the analogy of the relationship between the seven colors of the rainbow and the seven musical scale notes." Hunt based his theories on the relationship between notes, colors, and perfume on the "cosmic vibration scale" described in his book and which consists of sixty-two octaves of vibrations of those sounds.

Although not conclusive and certainly not specific enough to help you with your leapfrogging to discernment through frequencies, these documents should at least pique your interest into considering that I might be right. Honestly, the only way I can help you ferret out what sounds mean exactly harkens back to the other approaches: personal experience, feedback, and a healthy belief system. However, learning to feel/sense megahertz is more faithful a reading then just using colors.

I refer to these following concepts in my home-study course and book, *Happy Face Theory: Indigo Wisdom for Kids and Grown-Ups*. For example Itzhak Bentove, scientist, inventor and mystic, individualizes five resonance systems in the internal human body.

1. The heart/aorta system pumps the blood from the heart to the aorta, producing inside the skeleton a stationary wave of 7 Hz that causes an imperceptible movement in the body.
2. In reaction to this movement, the cranium makes the brain oscillate and produces acoustical waves of 1,000 Hz that reverberate in the brain itself.
3. The same acoustical waves activate other stationary waves in the brain's third ventricle (12,000 Hz) and lateral ventricle (4,000 Hz).
4. The sensorial cortex is stimulated by the stationary waves of the cerebral cortex. These frequencies collect in the intervals of audibility.
5. A pulsating magnetic camp is produced in each hemisphere of the brain.

Bentove also individualizes the fundamental brain frequency to be 4,000 Hz, the skull to be 2,250 Hz, the body's length at 375 Hz, the trunk and the head at 750 Hz, and the heartbeat at 2,000 Hz. Still other sounds relative to the internal body derive from the various systems: blood circulating in the veins and arteries, the workings of the nervous system, breathing and other sounds produced by the heart beating, and bone movements, to name a few. All these collect in the recess of the audible frequency, and we can hear them internally. As early as 1920, biofeedback instruments had been used to evaluate and heal. These instruments register the brain waves at intervals from 5 Hz to 22 Hz, and researchers have divided them into four different states of consciousness. The states are similar to those referred to in the dream and meditation or creative processes:

1. Beta Waves, with a frequency between 13 and 22 Hz and accompanying the cortical activity of thought. Beta Waves

give us our relative understanding or perceptions of the external world.

2. Alpha Waves, with a frequency between 8 and 12 Hz. These occur when a person is normally awake and in a state of total relaxation or meditation.

3. Theta Waves, with a frequency between 4 and 7 Hz, are produced while we sleep and in more profound meditative states.

4. Delta Waves, with a frequency between 0.5 and 3.5 Hz, are typical to sleep.

All these frequencies and many others are referred to as the natural vibrations of the human body.

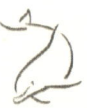

Chapter 13

Color Interpretations

Interpreting colors presents another enigma.

Being a psychic and clairvoyant is an advantage in interpreting colors, but you can still develop an understanding of the Aura without these characteristics. It only means that in seeing a certain color, with the added gift of clairvoyance you immediately know what the color and so on indicate. No one sees, perceives, or emits the same exact hue of colors. This one is really the most complicated of all of the tools of interpretation because it varies based on culture, previous lives, present life of the reader, and the subject. For example, upon reading an astral vision inside someone's Aura, I asked him to describe his visual and emotional experience while under a guided meditation. He was visiting another planet. The colors of that planet were reflected in his Aura, according to my psychic eyesight. We both saw a certain shade of brown, but I didn't ever remember seeing that shade of brown on this planet in this lifetime. I had to go deep into his former lifetime to understand the meaning of that brown for him in particular. After having discussed these color hues with him, and relating them to some of his psychological difficulties in that life and linking them with his unfinished karma in this lifetime, we were able to discern the profound and real meaning of that particular hue, compared to what the standard charts tell us.

I cannot give you the same color grid that I use, because I operate on a strange color system that seems to me from a totally different planet. Therefore, I've formulated a system for you that seems to combine a little of everything I've read and heard from my modern-day students. I still don't know where I developed my personal insights except that my mother's guidance, while helping me to sort out colors and their meanings, exposed me to many theories so that I might check them against my individual and autonomous perception. Another curious observation made by a UFO researcher was that I've been contacted by what he believes to be the ATLANTIS consciousness. If so, I'm not aware of it. But it could be another possible explanation for my unaccounted-for color perceptions. They compare to nothing in or on any of the charts I've ever read, books I've ever read, or color comparisons from other psychics with whom I've been involved, such as in the study of Tibetan medicine.

Ever since I was little I have seen hues and colors that I have not seen on this Earth plane. I know that I have lived many, many lifetimes in many different cultures. I also suspect that, along with the fact that many shamans say I was an Atlantis inhabitant, all this information has remained with me. I always remember seeing colors, from birth, and simultaneously knowing what these colors meant. (This possibility is supported by Madam Blavatsky's documents on theosophy, which state that all present material-form earthlings were from Atlantis.) For this reason, imposing upon you what and how I see would not be fair.

Gradually, in my childhood, I came to understand that I had either evolved into feeling frequencies or I was already there. When I force myself, I can transform these frequencies into color. In particular, I do this when I am teaching for those who need validation of their visual perceptions. All of this is impossible to understand until the day E.T. comes and explains it to me. I don't worry about it; I just do it, as I do when performing healing practices.

I have studied color interpretations from other cultures and have compiled a list for you of some of those. In addition, I've given you a more detailed color list that emanates from my years of experience teaching children. This could really be called the Kids' Chart. Whether you settle with one or combinations of all, undoubtedly it's because of your background, your past and present lives included. I introduce you to various understandings taken from other philosophies, and then you can decide how you see them and what you see in them. In this way I hope that you can incrementally rediscover your innate psychic capabilities.

The important element is the final interpretation. If we are exactly in unison on the interpretation, then we have succeeded in achieving the real end goal of color interpretation.

When first studying Tibetan medicine, our teacher was leading us in a cleansing meditation, a practice that all Tibetan physicians perform daily. We were told to concentrate on the colors or lack of color that we saw in our own auric body while meditating. Then our teacher checked our Aura to see if he saw the same thing. When he came to me, we always saw different colors but the identical interpretations. I realized that I should not become intrigued enough by another culture to abandon or have doubts in myself. You do the same. *Your color visioning is yours*, whether you actually see a color or you get a message or thought process that whispers to you the name and state of that color.

Now that I've presented you with this paradox, I'll give you some guideline charts. Follow the explanations in exactly the way I tell you. Choose and develop meanings for these according to trial and error on your part, feedback from subjects, and feedback from your own life.

From a Tibetan Tantric Point of View

Earlier in the book I said that a supreme drop (*tigle/chenpo*) exists that is located in the center of our heart chakra. When stimulated and activated by wisdom winds (*yeshe llung*), our mind and its energies become conducive to enlightenment. When we are enlightened, we eliminate suffering. This drop has a five-colored glow because it contains the pure essence of the five elements. This essence flows around our body always in these color hues and is visible in the various layers of our Aura (Lha).

This Aura can have many different colors according to our dominant chakra energy, emotions, and state of health. The Aura can be seen expanding and becoming more intensely colored when a person experiences good health, positive energy, and positive emotions. The Aura retracts under opposite circumstances.

According to Ngalso tantric self-healing, the Aura, when influenced by negative emotions, produces different dirty auric colors:

- Jealousy and fear produce a dirty green Aura.
- Pride and miserliness produce a dirty yellow or brown Aura.
- Anger and hatred produce a dirty blue or red Aura.
- Ignorance produces a gray or black Aura.
- Negative energies produce dark auric colors.

As we progress in the tantric self-healing practice, our Aura gradually becomes purer and we develop

- Rejoicing and courage, which produce a pure crystal-green Aura.
- Generosity, which produces a golden Aura.
- Love, which produces a pure blue Aura.
- Contentment, which produces a pink Aura.
- Wisdom (spirituality), which produces a pure white Aura.

According to Tibetan tantric medicine, the colors connected to the various chakras in descending order from the skull to the area of the sexual organs are

- White
- Red
- Blue
- Yellow
- Green

Different colors reflect different attitudes, moods, and energy patterns. Although you can generally identify what certain colors reflect, you must keep in mind that there are many shades of yellow, green, and the rest.

Another interesting discipline is the Egyptian culture. The ancient Egyptians formulated the doctrine of correspondence between colors and the threefold human constitution. It shows that the human being comprises differing layers of consciousness or planes of being, and possesses a separate vehicle for expressing each of these vis-à-vis the physical, etheric, astral, mental, and spiritual bodies. Each mode of consciousness related in some particular way to the three primary colors—red, yellow, and blue—symbolizing the corporal body (physical-etheric), the soul (astral-mental), and the spirit (spiritual consciousness), respectively. From this trinity emanates the secondary or complimentary colors such as orange, green, indigo, and violet, and by blending these seven major rays together with black and white, all other colors are obtained.

When the Tibetans refer to the colors of the chakras of purity, they refer to the strongest and vibrant version of that color. It is considered by them to be auspicious—what decorators call Chinese blue, Chinese red, Chinese yellow, Chinese green, etc. When we see someone's Aura, we are basically stripping down all their defenses—habits, stereotypes, manners, and pretenses—and looking into their true nature.

Therefore, when you learn to see the Aura well, you can verify it for yourself, by concentrating on certain thoughts while watching your Aura or telling people what their thoughts are when you see their Auras.

People usually have one or two dominant colors, as we previously stated. These are colors or auric pairs, and often are the person's favorite colors.

In addition to dominant colors, the Aura reflects thoughts, feelings, and desires that appear like flashes or clouds or flames, usually farther away from the head. For example, a flash of orange in the Aura indicates a thought or desire to exercise power and control. Orange as a dominant color is a sign of power and generally indicates the ability to control or influence people.

Since the colors of the Universe are well defined in the color wheels that artists use, you can use them as guides. Before you do, I suggest memorizing what I call the *color duo* or *color pairs*. Learn these color pairs, or auric pairs. They are not random combinations but are the best representations of what we see with our naked eye here on Earth. Therefore, these combinations are simple and basic to use, as for reading Auras, because our culture is more conditioned to vibrations.

Occult science teaches that the Central Sun emanates great vibrator rays or wave lengths of light, termed the *seven major vibrator rays*, from which spring the seven main types of human mentalities and temperaments. In order of degree these frequencies and mentalities are as follows:

Violet	Spiritual power
Indigo	Intuition
Blue	Inspiration
Green	Energy supply
Yellow	Wisdom
Orange	Health
Red	Life

Many of the disciplines that refer to visualization of colors speak first of the basic seven colors of the rainbow, exactly in the hues to which Easterners are more conditioned. However, one thing is true of all of the styles and color perceptions: understanding their significance, regardless of what chart you follow, takes time and practice.

Color Duo / Pairs Chart

We can follow this basic chart as we follow all the pure colors of the rainbow monochromatic colors. This table also applies to the intermediate colors. For example, yellow-green as seen by children always gives a pink-violet Aura.

- Red gives turquoise Aura; turquoise gives red Aura.
- Orange gives blue Aura; blue gives orange Aura.
- Yellow gives violet Aura; violet gives yellow Aura.
- Green gives pink Aura; pink gives green Aura.

I have found these color combinations to be consistent in my experiments with teaching children to see Auras in my Baby Playgroup preschool centers and in English yoga/meditation classes for junior high schoolers. They all confirm having seen these color combination pairs. I trust the visualization of children because they are more spontaneous and less inhibited than adults. Having researched the colors that Tibetan clairvoyants see, I can attest that the majority of these color hues and their interpretations seem to coincide with those interpretations of the Occidental children from my research focus groups. I maintain that these seem to be the best indications of colors for our society.

Look at Nature and you will undoubtedly agree with the kids. When the average child looks at a red bird, he sees turquoise body parts. Goldfish are always reflected with a blue hue. Sometimes you see an alternative color in nature. Auric sight is not playing games with you. It's a secondary nature color; when a flower grows on a tree, it rarely is any other color than violet, pink (purple), or red, because green leaves surround them. I learned this from the children in all their simplicity.

You probably already understand the basic colors that compose the color spectrum. But there is more: each of these seven great rays is divided into many subhues; the violet ray, for example, proceeding from the shorter to longer wavelength, is divided into heliotrope, amethyst, orchid, royal purple, wisteria, and lavender. In addition to these, science admits to many rays that are invisible to normal physical sight, as, for example, ultraviolet rays. (They are, however, visible to shamanic sight.)

Color Chart Developed by Children

The following section synthesizes information from my teaching sessions and research conducted in Italy, Egypt, and the United States. For these colors, the children collectively indicated them and interpreted their indications as follows.

Meaning of Clean Colors

Purple: Indicates spiritual thoughts, heightened spiritual awareness, self-esteem, and high ideals. Purple is rarely a strong point in the Aura. It appears only temporarily, something like a cloud or flame.

Light Purple: People who have a refined or polished spiritual nature. It indicates work in progress. These people are actively working on the balance of each aspect of their lives (personal, spiritual, professional), their attitudes, and accepting their existence and the existence of others.

Mid-Dark Purple: Teachers of their chosen spiritual path. They may be working on a few issues of balancing, but for the most part they are patient, kind, and willing to go out of their way for people.

Blue: A balanced existence, life-sustaining, transmitter of force and energy, relaxed nervous system. Spiritual searchers, people with that "I know there is something more to life" feeling.

Vibrant Blue: Pride, adoration, dedication. A subject with any shades of the lighter blues is generally beginning his or her spiritual quest—not a metaphysical quest but a journey that will fill in the missing pieces of current existence, such as that found in some religions like philosophies of the Buddhist Tantra, Vedic scripture, Gnostic scriptures, Egyptian scriptures, and so on.

Darker Blues: Typically indicate the subject has found his or her spiritual path and is continuing education in the chosen realm.

Dull Blue: Taking life for granted, being too content, perhaps appearing selfish, narrow-minded, arrogant, or self-righteous. Many traits also accompany religious zeal, such as self-righteousness, dedication, pride, adoration, and worship. These variations are usually indicated by some shade of blue.

Strong Blue: This color in the Aura seen by children always indicated people who were relaxed, balanced, and survivors no matter what situation life presents to them. Blue thoughts help relax the nervous system and bring about a balance of the mind, peace, tranquility, and harmony. For example, in a group of schoolchildren in Italy, after a meditation a young girl started to cry, asking me if I could predict if her father was near her. Asking what exactly she meant as being near, she said he was dead and wanted to know if I saw him in her Aura. I asked her how long her father had been dead because I did not see a deceased person in her Aura, but one alive. She said seven years. Herein lies the problem. It was not the fact as to whether

her father was dead but the fact that at thirteen years old, she still had not made peace with or accepted the so-called passing away of her father. I had the other children in the classroom meditate on her, visualizing the strong color blue for peace and reconciling the fact that her father was not present. Her sobbing stopped, and the children in the classroom all hugged each other for the remainder of the period. In a room that was otherwise chaotic and filled with hyper-nervous energy, blue-green maintained an Aura of peace and tranquility. (P.S. I told the child that she should no longer harbor this feeling inside of her and to insist on discussing the problem with her mother and to consider continued psychological therapy and honest, forthright conversation with her mother for this problem. The child seemed to have had the conversation. She discovered the real truth. Her father was alive but abandoned the mother when she got pregnant. I told the child to continue to meditate on this color, visualizing it and letting it help her to come to grips with the problem. After two weeks of this she seemed no longer to feel the weight of this torment and completed her delayed mourning.

Turquoise: A dynamic, highly energized quality of being and personality. A person who can influence others as a leader. A good organizer. Capable of doing many things simultaneously. By projecting the color turquoise, you can help another person get organized.

Green: Restful, calming, and indicative of natural healing capabilities. The stronger the green, the better the healer. It can also reflect a person who is reliable, dependable, and open-minded.
The bright greens going toward the blue spectrum indicate healing abilities.

Light Green Shades: Indicate the onset or potential for injury, and the subject should be cautious for the next few weeks.
Darker Green Shades: Generally indicate that the injury has already occurred and is in the process of healing.

Muddy Green: Jealousy, selfishness, possessiveness. Remember the expression, "Green with envy"? Green can also indicate self-doubt and mistrust.

Yellow: Joy, freedom, nonattachment, freeing or releasing vital forces. High mental activity. A yellow halo around the head indicates high spirituality. Detachment, one who can free and release vital forces. This color represents the joy and light brought by the sun and also denotes high intellect.

Pale Yellow: Around the hairline can indicate optimism, a high-spirited person, and thoughtfulness.

Golden Yellow: Spiritual wisdom denoting soul qualities.

Vibrant Yellow: Denotes intelligence, success, and determination.

Yellow Moving toward Orange: Awakening psychic abilities and clairsentience.

Muddy Yellow: Can reflect being overly critical, feelings of being deprived of recognition and being dogmatic, hypercritical.

Orange: Warmth, confidence, pride, and ambition, but without lust for power.
This orange ray comprises all shades of orange.

Dull Reddish-Orange: Denoting selfishness and pride.

Bright Clear Orange: A sign of health and vitality, the vital force, the energy of the sun. The Yogis call it the "soul of energy."

Orange-Yellow: High energy or a live wire, an active and vital person. People who dominate their peers by the sheer force of their vital qualities. They are people with a good smattering of pride, the kind of pride that is peppered with good common sense—just enough pride, which gives them the drive to succeed in bringing forth their message.

Dull Orange: A lack of warmth, but a strong desire for success and popularity. In general, this color can reflect an opening of new awareness—especially to the subtle realms (the astral plane) of life.

Muddy Orange: Emotional imbalances and agitation, excessive pride and flamboyance. It may also reflect worry and vanity.

Red: It's a very strong physical color, denoting strength, often a materialistic outlook on life. Materialistic thoughts and thoughts about the physical body, such as vanity, fear, and anger.

Remember the expression, "He was flame red with anger," or "burning with anger"? It's the color that affects the body's circulatory system.

Where red suffuses the Aura very heavily it shows a strong commanding nature, a magnetic personality. It's seen in pioneers and leaders of daring enterprises.

Bright, Clear Red: Generosity and praiseworthy ambition, a leader, a magnetic personality.

Vibrant Red: When seen in a clear and constant state, it represents fear or strong anxiety.

Dull Red: Generally represents anger. The deeper the red, the stronger the emotion.

Constant Dark Red: A consistent dark red indicates a violent nature and deceitful attitude.

Muddy Red: Can reflect overstimulation, inflammation, or imbalance. It may reflect nervousness, temper, aggression, impulsiveness, or uncontrollable excitement.

Cloudy Reds: Cruelty and greediness.

White: Indicates purity or protection. When white is detected in the outer layers of the Aura, it can indicate an area of the body that has been overenergized or overactive. White is the presence of all colors and thus indicates purity, simplicity, and directness of thought, Truth. When White appears strongly in the Aura it's often in conjunction with other colors, which is how you can know if it's an actual energy color or just a poor perception of the Aura. When white stands out as a color in the Aura, it's so definite and profound that you won't mistake it. It often reflects an awakening of greater creativity. Visualizations of white are usually of a faint streak somewhat fleeting, rarely constant.

Dirty, Muddy White: Artificial stimulation (drugs, alcohol) before it becomes a chronic ailment.

Pink: Achievement of a perfect balance between spiritual awareness and material existence. The most advanced people have not only a yellow halo around the head (a permanent strong point in the Aura) but also a large pink Aura extending farther away. The pink color in the Aura usually represents people who like a quieter life. It indicates compassion, love, and purity. Since it's a mix between being a good companion and having great, lasting devotion, nuns have a strong mixture of pink with heavenly blue in their mystic Aura, especially cloistered nuns. Love of art and beauty.
Muddy Pink: Immaturity, lack of truthfulness.

***Brown: It denotes industry—for example, a person who insistently strives to achieve in a business activity or series of activities. It's the ruling color of conventional thinking. Don't expect strong emotion from a "brown" person. It's also the starting point of ambition and power—material and commercial—and painstaking perseverance.
Brown Tinged with Green: The grabbing instinct, extreme selfishness and egocentricity.
Lighter Brown: Avarice, lack of confidence in oneself, the present situation, or the subject of the moment.
Dark Brown: Faultfinding and tendency toward deception, but in the form of exaggerated storytelling.
Dirty-Muddy Opaque Brown[15] Unsettling, distracting, materialistic, negating spirituality.

Gray: Lack of imagination, tendency to narrow-mindedness.
Heavy Opaque Gray: May be taken as showing meanness and dullness. Usually the plodding type who leaves no task undone because what they lack in imagination and fantasy they make up in unilateral fixation on the task at hand and are always the lone-wolf type.
Muddy Gray: A sign of a potential alcoholic or drug addict or an emotional codependent.
Dark-Muddy Gray: Dark thoughts, depressing thoughts, unclear intentions, presence of dark side of their personality.
Silver Gray (Streaked): A volatile, lively, unreliable personality. People gifted in all matters pertaining to movement, speech,

travel, and so on. Dabblers in all, but masters of none. Expect feebleness, inconsistency, and changeful moods where silver-gray predominates.

Platinum Silver: In a sort of twinkling effect, like a series of little lights. There are several meanings to this color. It's called *twinkle stars*, and often it's seen in highly fertile women and in women pregnant with twins. The children in general have seen this platinum silver around women and men as well who seem to possess a strong feminine tendency.

Black: Hatred, negativity, depression. When it appears in the Aura it's usually localized or appears as wisps drifting through it. In these cases the black spots resemble a hole or cavity that is eroding the Aura—As in the presence of extreme negativity due to externally imposed black magic spell, or chronic diseases.

Black also indicates a chronic, toxic dependency that not only carves black holes but also is found in an Aura that is beginning to separate from its physical body.[16]

These physical imbalances often show up in the Aura around or closest to the physical body. The location provides the clues. In the outer edge of the Aura, black holes indicate a trauma-induced illness such as seen in victims of child abuse or in substance abusers (alcohol, drugs, tobacco, etc.). Note that these holes can multiply and eventually erode the entire Aura, so that it's most important to be aware of purification or cleansing of these situations before they case nonkarmic or premature death.

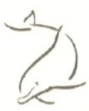

Chapter 14

Additional Aspects of Interpreting and Modifying the Aura

As you learn color interpretation, you should also become familiar with the location of the color and how the two relate.

The location, consistency, and clarity of colors within the Aura help to determine their full meaning. In the charts in the previous chapter, I gave you a broad indication of those meanings that apply to reading the Aura near the head, as around a person's halo. This is the first step in reading and interpreting the Aura.

As we have already noted, a vibrant and consistent yellow about the head indicates the positive aspect of yellow—a person's high spirituality and wisdom. But if just one of these parameters is modified, the meaning of the color can change. Alternatively, the same color around the chest could indicate high motivation, achieving personal spiritual growth, and willingness to help others to grow spiritually.

The Aura also reflects thoughts, feelings, and desires, which appear like flashes, clouds, or flames and are usually farther away from the head. These are desires not yet realized, desires in the stage of thought only. For example, one could want to have control over one's life. Consequently, you would see only a flash of the respective color.

Shape

In some cases you might see a dent in the Aura in a particular location. The Aura is not always perfectly egg shaped, as I indicated previously. It can be completely flat on one side, or S-shaped or distorted on another. This variation can occur for two reasons. The most common is an intrusion or interruption that has occurred to the subject.

Another reason for loss of auric energy could be that a person has suddenly walked past you and robbed you of some energy, and you had that feeling of the person suffocating you or intruding on your space. That intrusion into your Aura or space can interrupt your flow of energy.

Another situation causing a misshaped part of an Aura is living in the same household with someone who mentally wishes you harm or who is a negative character.

These situations leave you the most vulnerable. The people closest to you know and realize the fullest extent of your vulnerability and are those whose intentions you least suspect. Therefore, if they have negative intentions, you are most susceptible to their ill wishes, especially when in your own environment; when you are in your own home, you are more relaxed and normally let down your barriers and guard. These are common moments and places of attack for a great deal of black magic or voodoo potions. When a spouse wants to adversely control his or her partner, the black magic potions are placed in a beverage such as coffee, or they are in a powder-like substance placed in an anomalous object, such as a statue or vase. The magic is done by casting a spell and targeting that particular person in the house whom they wish to control. The operator places a powder in the object, hidden, and indicates chants to the client that ordered the spell to pronounce while the unsuspecting party is asleep. Recall the thirty-nine-year-old man I spoke about earlier who was a child of an alcoholic mother. When he came to me he was burdened with several black magic spells. A few months passed and he drank coffee that had a powder potion put in it without his knowledge. Months later, I discovered (psychically) powder in a statue in his bedroom. These have the most powerful effect on the person because, even when healthy, the target of the attack is in his or her environment naively feeling protected and disarmed, especially while asleep. In this situation, the spell can penetrate more quickly and easily and more profoundly, and since black magic always creates eventual death, the subject dies quicker than usual.

A commonsense philosophical version of this concept is as follows: my parents taught us to never, ever invite anyone into our home who was against us. Also, if we had to discuss business or have heavy negative discussions in the house, we needed to be very careful whom we invited into our home. If we were obliged to invite them, then we immediately purified the house after their departure. All this occurs because other people's thought energy projects onto the walls, ready for us to absorb the negativity in our most vulnerable moments.

In all these cases you might see a dent or hole in the Aura with an alternative color in it. For example, if the major color around the dent is green, it would mean an illness or upcoming illness in the umbilical chakra. However, if the color is lavender, it's more likely that an interruption of the energy field has occurred.

Consistency and Spikes

The parts of the Aura we have discussed in this book so far display consistent or primary energy patterns, such as the above-mentioned flashes. Layers within the pattern may change color, shape, or location, but this usually occurs gradually and over time. As a person's general attitude and health change, so does the primary energy field around the physical body.

Every action, physical or mental, creates energy and affects the Aura. Therefore, sudden emotions or thought patterns can generate instant energy pattern or peaks in the energy flow. This type of energy appears as a spike shooting out from one part of the body or a lightning bolt across the entire Aura. Emotions or sudden thought patterns may not last for a long period of time; the energy they produce is also quick and sudden.

Interpreting spikes is really no different from understanding consistent energy. Just keep in mind what spiking energy represents, and then apply the appropriate color interpretation to that sudden geometric appearance.

At this point you are ready to develop your own methods for reading Auras. You should use these indications only as a launching pad, not as set-in-stone rules and procedures. Don't become overly dependent on my system or the systems of others, because what works well for some does not work as well for others. Certain commonalties apply to all methods and their color interpretation, so pick and choose what works best for you.

Suppressing the Aura

Don't forget that certain things can reduce, muffle, or distort an Aura, such as fear, stress, anxiety, hatred, envy, jealousy, any other negative thought or feeling, physical discomfort, disease, artificial stimulation, drugs, and so on. All can cause a temporary increase in the Aura energy, such as when your body temperature rises when you are ill. ideally you can read the Aura before the inception of illness, to diagnose such a crisis and nip it in the bud.

Matching Color with Your Environment and Style of Dress

Clothes and the environment clashing with your Aura . . . what to do? Dull-colored clothes absorb your bioenergy rather than harmoniously enhance it. Many parapsychologists feel the reason that most men have a shorter life span compared to women is that they wear dull colors such as black, gray, or dark blue. Women wear much more colorful garments and change them frequently. Another interesting fact in Nature is that male birds are multicolored and more brightly colored compared to female birds, and male birds live longer.

Take a clue from Nature: don't wear too much black or gray. It will tire you quicker, make you look much older and age quicker, and also pull down your mood—especially wearing gray, black, or brown. At the minimum, try to cultivate color awareness that allows you to use colors to help alter a mood or thoughts in your mind. Perform a little do-it-yourself color therapy every day by learning the predominant colors of your Aura and matching the vibration frequencies of your clothing with your body and mind to create a new state of harmony. It's like tuning a musical instrument. Without tuning, all you can make with the instrument is noise rather than harmonious melody. Follow the suggestions below to achieve the desired effect.

Match Your Strong Points

Find the dominant colors in your Aura and attempt to match your surroundings or clothes with your Aura. Redecorating your home to achieve a better match can result in a positive stimulation of our psyche and will help to promote our well-being in many aspects. According to what Nature does to stimulate use, we should use auric color pairs aiming for such a match. For example, if your Aura is predominantly green, you should use green as well as a light pink in your decorations or apparels.

Amplify Your Aura

Match your surroundings to the frequencies of your thoughts. *Frequencies of thought* means that if you think about relaxing your mind (a blue thought), blue surroundings can amplify your thought. Note that when you come out of the house in the morning and the sky is perfectly blue, you feel relaxed before you have to think about anything else. The reason is that any thought in the direction of relaxing the mind is assisted by the blue vibration of the sky. When the sky is gray, you have depressing thoughts before you even notice it. Blue jeans are very popular because they help us achieve a relaxed mind. Promoting brown jeans may prove to be less lucrative.

The fashion all over the world in the last decade seems to be dress totally black. This mania, which started in Italy, is very risky to our society and its harmony, because it's creating more and more depression, with stronger feelings of being blocked in our lives and seeing nothing but obstacles. I've noticed that the people who continuously wear black in Italy are risking and have been losing the depth and width of their Auras. One strange phenomena is that high-fashion designers for years have been trying to reintroduce color into fashion, and it's very difficult to bring color use back into mode. A few years ago, a friend from the States came with me to Italy and asked me who had died because he thought that all the men and women were in mourning. Actually when I first went to Italy in the mid-1990s, I felt an overall gray atmosphere emanating amid the people that gave me a psychic sensation. People in the streets had tinges of gray in their faces.

They did not smile. They even had that facial expression as though their faces dropped to the ground. Subsequently, I discovered that liver disease and hair loss were rampant in Milan; mostly everyone was wearing black every day.

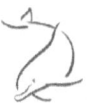

PART 2

Tantric Explanations

Tantric Lha, the Aura, Tibetan Somatic and Folklore
Medicine, Shamanic Secret Rituals as They Relate to
Blocking Black Magic, and Maintaining a Purified Aura

Chapter 15

Some Additional Facts on the Lha and Tibetan Medicine

Before reading this section, which is intended to enlighten you on the philosophies surrounding the Aura, it's best that you acquire some additional understandings of Tibetan medicine and some of its terminology. Consider it a crash course on dharma.

Tibetan medical science is a complete holistic system and philosophy that totally revolves around the psychological aspects of Homo sapiens as the root of all illness and disturbance. It's a curative system that considers the human body in its totality: mind, body, and spirit, not just as a single piece or part. Synergy and interdependence are key words in the philosophical and healing aspects. Modern traditional medicine addresses only the physical aspects.

The basic structure of Tibetan medicine is the mind. A little white ball and a little black ball represent the mind. The mind is analogous to a geometric expanse, space. Like all mass, space is limited in potential and light. The original nature of the mind is clear, and its capabilities are to be all-knowing, conscious of all things. In the mind resides the seed of Buddha or the Seed of Illumination, Wisdom. Our mind has no beginning; it travels without a sense of time. Given that it knows no nor does it possess a sense of time, it travels without beginning and without end until the future without end. (See the chart on Natural Intrinsic Nature and the Life/Death Cycle Chart on page 61 and 85). That is why shamans and clairvoyants have difficulty as children learning to sense physical time and are often disoriented or often can be off in their timing when making predictions. There is no time in that dimension. It's all now, the present.

This lesson in fact was one of the most difficult ones for me to learn during my various shamanic teachings. Zeroing in on the exact time sequence of a particular prediction that would satisfy the three-dimensional aspects of this Earth only comes with trial-and-error practice in the three dimensions. Things are very different and abstract there—with 7 times 7 times 7 times 7 times 7 times 7 times 7 dimensions, at least.

Second, understand that according to natural medicine, all of our health problems are—as the Tibetans call them—imbalances that begin in the mind. The implication is that all the origins of our illness or imbalances begin with psychological difficulties.

The physical and spirit bodies are divided, and they respond to chakras and channels. Each in turn corresponds to a particular color.[17] Since we have already learned that color is a frequency, let us call it ultraviolet rays.

Certain ignorances or "poisons"[18]—or as they call them, "defilements"—represent causes and conditions: they created illnesses on both levels, mind and body, that then correspond to the actual three zones and five chakras of the body.

Ignorance resides in the head (crown); attachment in the throat chakra; anger is in the heart chakra; pride and greed in the umbilical chakra; jealousy and desire (sexual as well) are in the secret Chakra. It's said that fear is the poison that engineers our body/chakra train—that is, fear of death or impermanence. Only when we overcome this fear of death will we begin to eliminate all our other ignorances. In fact, I address this problem with a solution in my book *Happy Face Theory*. Fear and sex, wrote Sigmund Freud, are the principal problems of all our physical and mental difficulties; Tibetan medicine agrees with Freud, saying that the reproductive organ is the treasury of all our energies. In as much as that desire produces dissatisfaction in the mind, especially when not fulfilled, unless we try to become self-actualized we experience a lot of discontentment and little gratification or satisfaction—constantly driven by our fears and desires. (See the Natural Intrinsic Chart on page 61.) Tantric sex books indicate that sex must be performed for the correct reasons: mutual love and reciprocal joy and energy through positive sharing. Sorry, you one-night-standers. Sex is to be performed with the correct partner, your love partner, in the correct frequency in order to give mutual pleasure. It's not to be a frivolous experience; otherwise, excessive desire can drive us to psychological difficulties, such as in the extreme case of a nymphomaniac or as an obsessive or unscrupulous out-and-out debaucher such as Don Juan, the womanizer who was damned for his immoral ways. Sexual fetishes or indiscriminate sex is a mental illness that leaves one prey to venereal diseases. The chain effect is simple; when one does not mend one's ways morally nor cure the physical disease in time it can become chronic and eventually have an impact on the mind and create dementia. This outcome usually happens in the case of an immoral chronic sexual extremist, primarily because the practitioner is angry and filled with hatred. It's not that they enjoy sex; it's because they hate and want to destroy and obliterate the world and in particular the opposite sex.

———————The Chakras and the Corresponding Physical Aspects

Chakras	Functions Regulated by Them	Color
Crown (head) (Ignorance, stupidity, fear, confusion)*	Brain and sensorial organs	White
Throat (Jealousy)*	Digestion and taste	Red
Heart (Anger, hatred)*	Memory	Blue
Umbilical (Pride, greed)*	Regeneration of organs; generation and maintenance of cell development	Yellow
Secret (Attachment and desire)*	Reproductive system and functions	Green

*These humors are rarely found in the single pure state. Therefore, combining possible humor types, the total possibilities are seven personalities—three pure, three mixed, and one combo with three humors.

———————

Each person has a different constitution or anatomical psychic makeup. They consist of either one or a combination of the three basic characteristics or humors. From these humors, a physician and tantric shaman can identify potential weaknesses or illnesses. Each humor corresponds not only to personality types but also to physical features that are too lengthy to mention in this work. For the sake of Aura healing, however, I've listed a few of the personality descriptions.

Since it very difficult and rare to find a single humor type, it increases the chakras and residence (zones) of potential illnesses.

When there is equilibrium between the three humors, one with another, we enjoy good health. To achieve this state, we need to be free from ignorance.

Biodynamic and Psycho-Physical-Emotion of the Humors

Humor	Sample Personality Type	Location of Potential Imbalances
Wind (*Llung*)	Nervous, fast, dark hair, short, unstable mind	Upper third of the body
Bile (Dul)	Ambitious, brown-blonde, medium height, egotistical, strong foot odor	Middle third of the body
Phlegm* (Badken)	Slow, externally calm, blonde, tall, very lucky, often rich, long life.	Lower third of the body

*On the lighter side, I imagine a lot of Tibetan mothers running around trying to find a male phlegmatic personality type for their daughters because it's said that the "phlegmies" have a propensity of great wealth.

These humors are manifested by one of three of the Samsara earth elements: water, air, and fire. The first energies that are manifested are two opposite energies: fire and water; their interaction produces air.

Corresponding elements Table

Water	Phlegm	Material
Fire	Bile	Energy
Air	Wind	Mind, including psychosomatic diseases

An example of the imbalance cycle is as follows: "I" imbalance is a wind problem, nervousness. First one manifests too much desire stimulated by fear, leading to throat or voice disorders. Anger is manifested as a heart problem. Pride is manifested in the colon or intestines. Excessive fear or excessive sexual desire creates craziness, which leads to close-mindedness (obtuseness) and results in stupidity.

Tibetan medicine, relatively unknown in the West, is a multifaceted approach to health that has been adopted right from its time of origin. Of the utmost importance in Tibetan medicine, as in all Oriental medicine, is for the physician to acquire impeccable diagnostic skills. Disorders or symptoms are known to have their origins first in the mind, and then they reside in the body. The mind and body have the categories of gross body, subtle body, and very subtle body. After having identified the cause of an illness, a Tibetan physician then begins to choose the mode(s) of therapy. Treatment takes the form of a single mode of treatment, such as acupuncture or herbal medication, and other supportive therapy such as massage, bloodletting, moxabustion (heat therapy), or color and gemstone therapy, and so on, as well as weighted reliance on patient feedback and interaction. When all else fails, physicians look to esoteric gurus of Aura or Lha to intervene.

First, here's some additional understanding of how a physician categorizes a human problem, because there is very little division between the theories of Tantric medicine and tantric Aura healing. Above all, both types of practitioner encourage the client to assume responsibility for one's own health.

Theoretically, Tibetan medicine is based upon elemental materialism. However, for all practical purposes, health is evaluated in terms of the major organs and systems in the body. Because Tibetan physicians have to rely upon themselves as diagnostic tools, they have devised a system of reference known as the three-humor models in order to arrive at a correct diagnosis and treat the client. There are four main origins of illness: karmic with 101 disturbances, subcategorized into 404 maladies for each 101—to be treated only by an esoteric healer (spiritual medicine); mental, with 404 disturbances—healed by a combination of spiritual and somatic medicine; humoral, with 404 disturbances, which are illness of this lifetime—curable via somatic medicine with or without the need of a spiritual healer; and miscellaneous, 404 minor illnesses that may or may not require an active cure, because in these cases the body can heal itself (example: a cold or a bruise from a fall).

When the physician diagnoses a disorder such as wind, the first humor, he generally refers to any of the following: a functional or even organic disorder of the nervous system, the heart, or large intestines, a functional circulatory disorder, and psychological problems. Psychotic disorders are not included, however, as they are classified separately. A physician who talks about a bile disorder could be referring to a general infection or inflammation, or one specifically of the gall bladder, liver, small intestines, or the lungs. Similarly, in talking about a phlegm disorder, the physician is basically referring to a noninflammatory and often chronic condition of the stomach, spleen, or kidneys.

Treatment is based on symptoms present and the clinical picture arrived at from urine analysis, pulse taking, physical examination, and questioning. A number of factors like the severity of the disorder, age of the client, season, location of the disorder, the client's digestive power, and the presence of complications also determine the actual type of treatment indicated.

The ideal form of treatment according to the medical texts is a multifaceted one. When the client and physician both have the time and facilities, treatment can be highly elaborate and graduate, waiting for an evaluation of the physical response from the patient, The first line of treatment is *nutrition and behavior therapy* that normally supports the second line of treatment: *medication.* Several types of oral medications are graded and used according to definite clinical information. Oral medication is supported by therapies such as oleation, emetics, purgatives, mild enemas, suppositories, nasal inhalants, and washes. When these fail to correct a disorder, or when the disorder is severe and chronic, the third line of treatment known as *external therapies* is recommended. External therapy is massage, hydrotherapy and fomentation, acupuncture, moxabustion, and vein section supported by surgery.

Disorders accompanied with major physical symptoms of abdominal discomfort and distension is a condition when overstressed with functional problems of the sympathetic nervous system could result in a wide range of diffused symptoms. The first step is to deal with the symptoms, particularly the physical ones, with oral medication supplemented by nutrition and behavioral therapy. The strategy is twofold: first to remove the symptoms, and second to intentionally concentrate pathological activity in the gastrointestinal region. Once the external symptoms are reduced, the diet and behavior are corrected, and the pathological activity is localized in the gastrointestinal region, a mild enema followed by a moderate or severe one is given so that the pathological activity of wind is expelled from the body system. Oleation therapy and massage are recommended to improve blood circulation and provide energy to the body. Oleation therapy is particularly effective in improving the digestive system. At this point, if the client still complains of symptoms like backache, numbness, palpitation, and so forth, it's time to consider Hor moxabustion, which is a heated medicated pack applied on certain points. Heated packs are extremely effective for instant relief and widely recommended for wind disorder causing pain, swelling, and numbness. In case Hor moxabustion does not alleviate the problem, moxabustion using a more concentrated heated Artemisia cone is recommended. I have personally found that the Nepalese Artemisia species is the most effective and gives immediate results, but it should never be used in a closed, non-aerated room because of its toxicity in excessive doses.

Once these symptoms are totally controlled, the next step is to restore the vital body functions, which may have been disrupted by treatments such as enemas. Medicated wines and medicated oils are indicated as vitamins to strengthen the body and assist in the proper functions of its systems.

Energy and Nervous Systems

The human being, according to Tibetan medical philosophy, comprises a number of psychological units—sensory, mental faculties, and biological. They are known as the three humors, and they have seven constituents or systems. At the gross level, the body functions in relation to the activities of the three humors, whose normal functioning are vital for good health. However, at the subtle level, there is an intricate relationship between biological activities and mental activities. For instance, repeated anger can cause or provoke the disturbance of the flow of energy in the nervous system, which in turn causes pathological conditions in the nerves themselves. While the Tibetan physician is aware of this subtle relationship, the Tantric practitioner is concerned with the power of the mind over the body, primarily involved in the study of the three humors or physiological processes and how they influence and affect the functions of the organs and systems of the body.[19]

The fields of anatomy and physiology of the body in Tibetan medicine include the knowledge not only of gross organs and systems but also the circulatory and lymphatic systems. There are eleven main organs, and as in Chinese medicine, they are divided into positive or solid and negative or hollow organs. Each positive organ has a functional relationship with a negative organ. For instance, the liver, a positive organ, is responsible for the production of blood while the gall bladder, its supportive (negative) organ, is responsible for the storage of bile, a byproduct of blood. The organs in turn form and support the functions of the seven constituents such as the muscles, circulatory, and adipose tissues. From ancient times, Tibetan physicians have identified ligaments, sutures, the lymphatic system, nerve plexus, fascia, adipose and vascular tissues, and mucus and synovial membranes.

According to Tibetan anatomical texts, three major energy pathways in the body carry out the functions of the three humors. The *black pathway* is the pathway through which blood flows, the *wind pathway* (blue) is the central and secondary nervous system, and the *white pathway* is the lymphatic system. However, in the explanatory Tantra that includes the section on anatomy and physiology, these three energy pathways are often referred to by the names of the three-Tantra pathways. The medical pathways are clearly distinct from those of the Tantra pathways. The Tantra channels are not physiological in a gross materialistic sense, in that they do not function actively in ordinary sentient beings. They only function when a practitioner achieves the Creation State of the yogi. Only the gross manifestations, the three medical manifestations, along with his cultivated psychic power are able to open them as a real structure. In the ordinary being, these are latent and only their gross manifestations, the three medical pathways, actually function in the body, as in cases of spirit possession, black magic, or karmic[20] causes.

According to ancient methods of Tibetan self-healing, NgalSo e Sowa Rigpa, illnesses are determined by an imbalance of the three primary energies (wind, bile, and phlegm) that constitute our psychophysical system.

Self-healing methods aim to rebalance the three energies that first manifest themselves in physical sickness. Self-healing works through meditation practice united with the recitation of a mantra, a specific regime of an alimentary diet, and appropriate behavior combined with aromatic herbs. Consequently you need to find out what your constitution and personality combinations are according to the Tibetan evaluation system. With this information, you can properly understand what foods are like medicine when ingested and what foods are like poison to your particular energetic base. For example, in the case of an imbalance of wind humor, you should avoid broccoli and, in particular, bitter-tasting vegetables. Even former president George H. W. Bush was against this great-tasting vegetable. Do you remember his public blooper about broccoli? He probably suffered a wind humor disorder. If you suffer from a bile imbalance, avoid cows' milk and any cow milk products (lactic acids). If you suffer from an imbalance of the phlegm humor, avoid spinach—Popeye not included.

The Human Body

Buddhists divide the human body into three parts: gross, subtle, and very subtle.

GROSS BODY (Life Energy of Gross Physical Body—Srog, the Densest Energy)

Body	Mind
1. The three humors: wind, bile, and phlegm	1. The five sensations: sight, hearing, smelling, tasting, feeling
2. The seven constituents or systems: chyle, blood, muscle tissues, adipose tissues. bone tissues, marrow, and regenerative fluid	2. Mental consciousness
3. The three excretory processes: feces, urinary, and perspiration.	

SUBTLE BODY (Life Span or Life Force—Tse; the energy that keeps us alive for a certain number of years; circulates through our Aura body)

1. The three Tantra pathways: right, central and left.	1. The three instincts or poisons: associated with hatred, desire and ignorance and emotions, in 80 subinstinct
2. Endocrine drops: the essence of lymph in the body.	
3. Blood essence and emotions.	

The subtle body is the core of our body and can be treated similarly to the physical body. It has five strata and five original colors; the secondary colors are "twin" colors. They can be considered first around the crown chakra; in order of closeness to the skull, yellow, blue, red, green, and white. This is the first area for a shaman to examine when investigating psychiatric and psychosomatic mental disturbances.

VERY SUBTLE BODY (Very subtle Lha)

1. Indestructible energy drop holding clear light—the mind that continues from one life to another	1. Mind of clear light

Note: In addition we have even more subtle astral bodies such as the dream body, the bardo body, and the illusory body.

An external imbalance of the elements can create an internal imbalance that affects the corresponding organs:

Table of Correspondence

Organs: Vital/Whole	Sense	Humor
Spleen/Stomach	Smell (Nose)	Phlegm
Kidneys/Bladder	Taste (Tongue)	Phlegm
Liver/Gall Bladder	Sight (Eyes)	Bile
Lungs/Colon	Touch (Skin)	Wind
Heart/Intestine	Hearing (Ears)	Wind

Tibetan medicine consists of two aspects: spiritual (more esoteric) and somatic (more traditional).

Both approaches are addressed in the Four Tantra (*gu-she*). Each volume discusses different aspects. The first part, the *Root Tantra*, consists of 6 chapters and addresses the principles that are the main essence of Tibetan medicine. The next volume, the second gu-she, is called the *Explanatory Tantra* and is divided into 31 chapters. It begins with the explanation of the formation of life and ends with the death process, discussing elements along the way such as diet, therapy, ethical codes of the practitioner, and causes and classifications of illness. The third gu-she, the *Oral Transmission Tantra*, consists of 92 chapters and relates to the practical experience of the student and the causes, nature, treatment, and classification of illnesses. The final gu-she regards various illnesses and is subdivided into those involving sensorial organs, whole organs, hollow organs, pediatrics, female, male, geriatrics, the poisons, and external injury. The last Tantra, called the *Last and Conclusion Tantra*, is divided into 27 chapters and covers subjects such as pharmacology, diagnosis, therapies, and so on—with a total of 156 chapters in all. The Tibetans categorize even what they call sections and sheets of these 156 chapters; there are 396 sheets and 39 sections.

The concept of the tantric teachings are not only transmitted by mystical manifestation of Buddha to those in a mystical state of purified karma and perception, but the teachings are themselves very mystical and spiritual. The underlying philosophical concept is called the Root Tantra of Kalachakra. Its purpose is much less material and more spiritual than the others are. The commentaries that came later, written by Tibetan scholars, are clarifications of Buddha's words. Their purpose is to help us purify the defilements of our body, speech, and mind as well as their imprints on our mental continuums. These defilements (see chart for list on page 169) or violations and imprints on our minds won't just go away by themselves. We have put into practice ways to receive empowerment and ripen our mind streams, and then we must receive an explanation of how to apply what we learn; it's called *liberating commentary*, the Kalachakra means wheel of time. (The Kalachakra diety which is represented by a wheel illustrates to particular aspects of an enlightened mind. When we learn the application it is referred to the liberating commentary) We can only attain realization of these understandings when we are complete and total practitioners of these theories and ways of living, which by some are referred to as the right view of the Absolute Truths. When we have accomplished this, we can enter the mystical kingdom of Shambhala.

The five great elements of the micro and macrocosm and their headquarters.

Astrological elements   **Kalachakra Tantra**

Organs

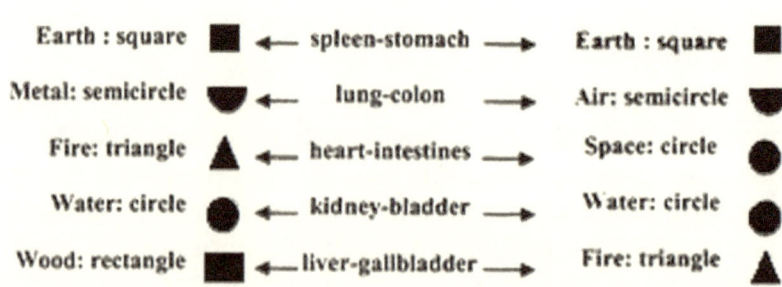

Astrological elements	Organs	Kalachakra Tantra
Earth : square ■	← spleen-stomach →	Earth : square ■
Metal: semicircle ▼	← lung-colon →	Air: semicircle ▼
Fire: triangle ▲	← heart-intestines →	Space: circle ●
Water: circle ●	← kidney-bladder →	Water: circle ●
Wood: rectangle ■	← liver-gallbladder →	Fire: triangle ▲

Shambhala is the only pure land situated in this Earth. Shaped like a giant lotus, having eight petals, it's surrounded by rings of snowy mountain ranges and is shielded from the outside world by its natural geographical composition and by supernatural forces. Some say it's fictional and some say they have actually seen it in physical form. Its inhabitants are born in this land because of pure karma, and they live according to high moral precepts in direct communion with the ultimate reality of Buddha or God. Being the inhabitants of the only pure land in this turbulent world, they lead a highly evolved spiritual life free from suffering and strife. They practice the highest Tantric teachings of the Buddha—the Kalachakra. This goal is the final goal of both somatic and spiritual (esoteric) Tibetan medicine—to lead many to liberation and enlightenment and eliminate Samsara (sufferings).[21] We complete our Samsara karmic sufferings via multiple reincarnations until we are yogi, living in Shambhala.

Both types of practice, medical and esoteric, rely on special gifts on the part of the practitioner, each different from the other. Both require certain permission or "caste structure" acknowledgment—a sort of karmic heritage traditionally handed to those "chosen ones" via a spiritual legacy or lineage accompanied by blessings and approved training and practices. These ceremonies increase the receptivity, satisfaction, and comprehension of listening and studying. They also increase the powers of the therapies applied to the patient under the guidance of that particularly designated god/goddess or divinity as their protector. When one receives these blessings, the therapy performed is much more effective because the practitioner is certain of transmitting only excessive *positive* energy. The esoteric practice is rarer and more difficult to learn and is connected to certain initiations and religious practices. Normally, medical practice evolves around and is based on the Four Tantras. People born to be healers must complete the study of the Tantra.

By now, you have probably come to realize that the importance and strength of a Tibetan healer is his or her spiritual motivation and diagnostic capabilities. In the way they must pay close attention to the supporting evidence regarding that patient as much as it consists of a conversation with the patient that allows for the physician to assess progress, pulse, tongue, ear, and eye reading, and a series of available therapies (somatic and spiritual). The physical healer and the esoteric healer both must study not only the philosophical aspects of their version of the Ars Medica but the esoteric and spiritual diagnostic and therapeutic cures as well. (The Shaman further undertakes study in alchemy and the physician continues study in pharmacology.) Of course, each one has a specialization, not to mention the village oracles who suck out illnesses with their mouth or produced protective devices from their mouth, sometimes in the form of gold necklaces, for example. All the specializations depend on this karmic lineage.

Negativity resides first in the Lha. The precepts of Tibetan medicine say that the emphasis is placed on the "nature of the human mind," and our conscience is the seat of the wind, eventually having an impact on the physical anatomy, as do the esoteric practices. Therefore, from both types of practitioners' points of view, the mind is the primary conscience, while the conscience of the body is secondary. This also includes the mind impressions that emanate from our parents' conscience and from the karma of our previous lives. Often, when in doubt, the physician has a diagnostic tool available, such as special forms of urinalysis. The guru has his clairvoyance and reading of the Lha at his disposal, for diagnostic purposes. Therefore, in Tibetan medicine the physician is usually the first one responsible for identifying and diagnosing when the symptoms are related to some outside influence of negativity. These practitioners know when to refer people to the guru/healer, whether he is a physician or one with special magical, metaphysical powers to identify and heal the aspects of the negativity.

It's indicated clearly in the study of medicine that there are 404 classified illnesses in the human body: 101 due to karma and 303 due to humors. A particular group is due to spirits who reside or attack various physical body organs; however, their first stop is always the Lha and chakras. The spirits then adversely impact our mental and psychological state. Some spirits are negative by nature, and some that are otherwise passive become vindictive when disturbed by defilements of our mind.

All psychological problems and mental sufferings come from our ignorance. This is the root of confusion. The less ignorant we are, the less the phenomena of these negative energies will affect us or leave us victims of their prey. When we harbor no ignorance, these spells cannot influence us. This is the point of view of Tibetan physicians as well as energy gurus. Therefore, the more faith we have, the more strength we gain to increase our immunity to these external causes. However, the influences often might remain within or outside our Aura and only slightly influence our mental, physical, or economic health. That is normally because we have not learned the necessary karmic lesson. (I often explain this to clients as that feeling of what we refer to as "for every ten steps forward we take, we are being pushed backward and losing nine steps.") An astute spiritual shaman might have to say, "No, not the time to help you yet." I have had several occasions when I gently had to decline transforming these invaders because the individual had not yet actively worked out the lessons they needed to learn from these obstacles. Most Westerners do not comprehend and accept when a person declines this type of assistance and insists on jumping from healer to healer until some charlatan charges an enormous figure to do nothing. Perhaps, that, too, is part of their karma, to get burned by the fire before they see the warmth of the light.

We address the mind in modern science as being that element that is situated in the brain. But Tibetan medicine visualizes the space reserved for the mind as very, very small. It's held and contained in the internal central channel, in a drop of extremely subtle, almost invisible material called the *Kua*, in the heart chakra.

To treat both types of negativity both practitioners must work on helping the client overcome his or her ignorance through a spiritual voyage. The more spiritual we become, the larger the seed or drop grows. That is why I try instructing those who ask me to "remove" (the correct term is "transform," but so many cultures incorrectly use the word "remove") negativity from them or the environment to try to find a spiritual path or spiritual educational system that feels comfortable to them. With spiritual practice and true compassion, this will aid in eliminating all further sufferings and no longer allowing purposefully imposed negativity to be absorbed. This is my goal in presenting you this book and my goal when one seeks my consultation. This should be the goal of all practitioners of the esoteric: to help create autonomous self-healing while we are guiding people on their passage, after having eliminated any and all negativity, regardless of its origins.

You might wonder why I have emphasized only wind or psychological problems in discussing Tibetan medicine. Of course, there are other types of disorders in Tibetan medicine too vast to address here. The reason I addressed the wind problems is that these imbalances indicate mental or psychological or psychosomatic problems, such as when one is attacked by negativity, imposed internally, externally, or otherwise. Wind is also pervasive, not stable, and dispersed throughout our nervous system.

The Lha is pervasive also; the two are linked and affected by the imposition of black magic or spirit possession. When black magic is pointed to a specific illness or chakra, of course, that illness is first manifested in the mind. It then pathologically, if we are in an extreme state of imbalance, renders adverse affects on the potential evil causes (spirits) created by mental contaminations. These spirits that are already inside of us because they reside in different organs become disturbed; at that point we can trace the contamination according to the specific potential organic disorders. Each disturbance is correlated to the headquarters of the disturbed spirit, such as when the Spirit that is housed in the liver is turned upside down by our actions, or through the direct imposed actions of others, our liver malfunctions. (Note: The shaman who decides to confirm this with a fresh urine sample will clearly see disturbances in either the second, fourth, or sixth "house" of the urine chart.) In turn, the sense organ, the eyes, which is the "door" or "flower" of our liver, or the ears or auditory canal that is the flower of our kidney, could be affected as well, and so on.

When black magic is not pointed to a specific chakra or type of illness (except in the case of an auto accident or death wishes), the organs that manifest a disease are always our weakest points that correspond with our humor type. The shaman works on these channels, which are connected to the nervous system, and all meditation and purification is performed through these channels. For example, I had a thirty-four-year-old male subject whose mother, at the suggestion of her physician, came to me to examine his energetic problems. The physician after two and a half years of psychiatric, herbal, and official medicine cures said to her, "We have done everything we could do; this case is the work for a faith healer." With this insight she contacted me and brought his medical chart. He was primarily classified with paranoiac phobia. He was afraid to go out and to be with people, refused to go to work and was convinced he was dying. According to the physicians his illness was psychosomatic. He continuously demonstrated a special type of psychobabble with little or no pathology. Upon examining him, his pulse, and his Aura, I found a problem with the hypothalamus. There was a definite hyperactivity that can create obsessive compulsive behavior. In addition, his Aura was detached due to his fear. The cerebral enzymes in the frontal brain that produce courage were also underactive and deficient. Further examination of the urine produced evidence in the second house, which is brought about by human witchcraft—or as the famous Spanish/Jewish/French shaman, director, and writer Alejandro Jodorowsky calls it, "psycho-magic"—and which produces extreme psychic wind and humor problems. In trance I noticed that there was also an article hidden in his automobile that was infused with a negative potion. First, I told the mother to examine the car well. She found in the recesses of the auto a very, very tiny doll stuffed with powder. I promptly destroyed it in the proper ritual fashion. I neutralized and operated on the very, very subtle wind channels as well as reattaching his Lha to his body. He improved within weeks and resumed going to work.

Another example of this phenomenon is the case history of a young woman approximately thirty-three years old. Prior to visiting me she had been in and out of hospitals, had been to many physicians, and had visited many faith healers. No one could determine the causes of her symptoms. Official medicine said she had a weakened kidney because she suffered from water retention. Her other symptom was a form of paralysis that left her unable to walk for two years. Not finding any causes for these symptoms when hospitalized, they pumped her up with cortisone injections, which only increased her symptoms. Upon examining her I found three pulses, which indicated spirit possession (of former lives and present life). She was still attached to her deceased father (unfulfilled mourning), and her Aura had completely detached, probably the result of heavy drug treatments for years. All her real estate properties were riddled with unhappy spirits. She had water retention of the kidney, constipation, and a knot at the base of her brain. I attributed most of her symptoms to negativity. Because, as previously explained, negativity often attacks the nervous system, it eventually travels from one organ to the next. In her case, the disease created a parabiotic suspension whereby it stopped the conductivity and excitability of the nervous system, thus creating paralysis or rigidity of the muscular system. After I immediately began working in trance at a distance in prayer first on the internal and external negativity and reattaching her Aura, she began to walk with assistance right away and in two to three days was walking unassisted—all this before I helped her father go into the celestial world and transform the agitated spirits residing in her various real estate properties. Now she is working on the stomach and constipation symptoms through karmic regression, doing some spiritual homework. She resumed a normal life in just three months' time, with the other symptoms gradually diminishing.

Remember that there are 404 categorized illnesses in Tibetan medicine, 360 spirits that can create interference, and an additional 1,080 types of mental interference. These interferences are the type that manifest illnesses. Shamans say there are eighty thousand evil causes of sufferance for sentient beings. Physicians and shamans both must be able to identify the causes before deciding on the therapy.

The most important human system for the purposes of purification against spirits is the circulatory system. This system is divided into the vein and arterial systems. The arterial system is the principal channel of the mind. It's this nervous system that constantly moves, just as the mind always moves. Neither system is fixed. For example, the mind is involved constantly with external sensations via our five senses. When we hear music, we perceive the sound; this is the mind that is operating. The conductor is the mind, and the mind's container or receptor is the mind itself and the nervous system. The transporter of the mind is the first stop for subtle effects of negativity. This sensation is called *Scepa*, the identifier of positive or negative input, and it reflects back to the interior mind and the exterior mind as that which it first perceived through the five senses.

Because this subtle or profound mind needs to be activated in order to be healthy, it flourishes in the arterial system. For this reason, we concentrate our meditations on this channel. This special type of meditation, however, is a little bit too advanced for this book. That is why I've given you all a simple mediation tool previously. In a later chapter I offer a visualization for blocking and protecting against negativity in a very simple abbreviated format. For the sake of clarity I explain here how complicated a shaman's work or my work can be when purifying people who come with damaged or severed Auras, because it's not a process and responsibility to be experimented with or taken lightly.

In spiritual science we speak about channels, the channels of wind. In reality a channel for wind does not exist, but it's the vehicle of the mind, the imaginary, because the mind flourishes through these blood channels, the arterial channels. The arterial system is the system that furnishes energy to the vital organs. They (twenty-four categories of channels) form, sustain, develop, and give nutrition to the cells. From there they go on to all the cells of the body. They then vitalize all the organs. When this fluid or liquid is interrupted by negativity, as happens with black magic, it first demonstrates its presence in the less subtle mind and then flows and adversely affects the subtle mind, which is in the central nervous system, then infects all the organs of our body.

This takes time, and the length of time before a practitioner arrives can prove fatal, depending on the person, the black witch's degree of force, who has invoked this and the spirit who invaded it, and the astrological aspects of the receptor. When we see people who have had problems with attacks on, or separation of, their Aura, it invariably manifests gradually in multiple manners but always indicates mind problems. As in the case of a trauma, such as an accident or other shocks, in which the Lha was separated, the person starts to regress to infancy, recuperates a little, and then if not healed often becomes a drug user. All these elements manifest in the mind. And when people are losing their Aura because of possession or black magic, they start to change their behavior drastically compared to their original character.

In the case of mental illness caused by spirit possession or Lha interruptions, no therapeutic medicine in the world can stop its deleterious effects. This is the exclusive work of a Shaman. If purification is not performed due to this toxin, the body does not absorb nutrients nor the three important foods required for a person to survive. The foods we require are of three types: material food, air, and spiritual food. We need all three for a healthy mind and body.

When there is interference from outside forces, we get ill and diseased. It's also true that too frequently imposed negativity, such as black magic, performed on the same person diminishes the vital energy. When this happens, one becomes weak and unable to combat day-to-day life in the same way as previously and mental confusion is augmented. In fact, without this strength, we often unconsciously seek that food that is bad for us instead of the food that is good for us. (For example, one runs away from a church, or the victim continues to pursue the person who put black magic on them, and has extreme difficulty in severing their relationship or thoughts of that person.) The victim, therefore, puts himself constantly in the hands of the same masters of evil (that which is bad for him) and runs away from the masters of good (those who are good for them). In these cases the only beneficial approach is (1) have it handled by a shaman and (2) after the shaman has finished, refurbish your three areas of nutritional needs. Go out and breathe in good, fresh air, and let it enter your lungs. Meditate. Change your environment or your behavior patterns. Have faith.

These channels and the previously mentioned five chakras form the larger chakra. These chakras are entry points for negativity. While concurrently damaging the mind, negativity enters one or eventually all of the five chakras and the corresponding organs or the individual's weak humoral points, the first stop for the physical illness.

Chapter 16

The Lha:
Its Secrets and Mysteries

The Lha is very similar to the Aura; it's called the second body of the human being, and it's a group of very subtle channels that to the psychic eye reflect like the light of colored glass—all of a natural, intrinsic nature.

There are five hundred channels in each chakra (gross and subtle), all connected and related. While an individual person can help heal her or his body by visualizing the colors of the chakras, a shaman works on the esoteric Lha to heal problems that arise from internal and external negativity. Since these chakras are interrelated, we ask the client, as a rule, to work on the physical aspects and needs of the prospective chakras, either by visiting a physician for support therapies or meditating and Aura visualization, or both. In the absence of this possibility, the shaman performs additional rituals to effect a cure via energetic thought pattern projection, which is considered to be absorbed from a seed of illumination within us and flows through our being. Then we use this force mentally to help the infected subject let his natural self-healing process begin by reorganizing the murkiness in the Aura—transforming it.

We have spoken about chakras and channels, and now we understand that these terminologies are used in both tantric medicine and tantric spirituality. We also understand the separate roles of the physician and the shaman.

The chakras are the fundamentals in which all of these channels are concentrated. These seven hundred principal channels for each of the five gross chakras with a total of seventy-two thousand more subtle channels that are reserved for the more elevated spiritual shamanic healing. One group is the brain, where the nervous system is concentrated. Another is the throat; another, the chest; another, the umbilical; and the last, the genitals. They are exactly the same zones as the spiritual chakras. It's important to understand at this point that the practice of spiritual medicine works on an imaginary chakra or zone. They really don't exist; you cannot touch them, so therefore we must create them mentally, giving them the specific colors we mentioned previously.

The Vital Channel (*Tse/Tza*) contains our Lha. This Lha is not stable, it's pervasive. The Lha Channel is the white channel; therefore, our nervous system is dominated by wind. The nature of wind, too, is pervasive, as it is connected to the lymphatic and endocrinology system, which, according to Tibetan medicine, is unstable. That's why negativity, black magic attacks by spirits, and absorbing negative emotional or sexual energy from others affects the mind or nervous system secondarily—because of its mutability. Meditating on the five colors of the five lotuses is the more complicated of the meditations to assist in healing. But remember we said that there are other villains to our health. They can be these 360 different spirits that create interference, and which can also damage, separate, and eat up our Lha with craters that eventually erode the Aura. These spirits and black magic work on your esoteric body, the Lha.

Negativity that cuts the Lha provokes changes on a mental level. The other consideration is in the case of traumatic separations that I mentioned earlier. In these situations, we realize that the Lha has been abandoned, not only with our third eye, but through a series of manifested specific symptoms.

Case History

Boy age eight years, six months. Living in the United States. Diagnosed as ADHD Syndrome. *Esoteric diagnosis:* Lha separated from body. Negative reaction and fear of being enclosed or suffocated. *Origins:* Former lifetime in Egypt. *Mother's objective:* Controlled gradual elimination of prescribed drugs, Ritalin in particular. *Esoteric objective:* Give him back his sense of security and eliminate his fears of abandonment. *Secondary objective:* Free his fears in order to release and recognize, without trepidation, his highly developed natural gifts of psychic sensitivity and artistic abilities.

After one week, the mother (a practicing nurse) reports that he no longer needed the meds. After two weeks he showed no symptoms of outbursts or temper tantrums, or any of the other manifestations that had accompanied ADHD. Oh yes, I forgot one thing. He had an argument with a playmate because he unknowingly read his thoughts and it was something that offended his chum. The boy explained these thought flashes as having heard the words. The mother knew that no words were verbalized but that her son was demonstrating telepathy. Since then, several similar accounts have occurred. The final phase of the therapy was to work with him proactively to realize this delicate capability and how to manage it. One of the ways we used was offering him children's handmade play toys with rice leaves from Egypt. One of the items was a pharaoh's boat. During one analysis of his Aura, I noted that he was once in peril on a boat and in danger of capsizing. I wrote and published a play methodology that increases attention skills and helps in eliminating fears not only for what some categorize as indigo, crystal, or rainbow children but which works well for all attention deficit syndromes. I also used this program in Cairo, Egypt, for special-needs children along with swimming with dolphins and beluga whales. It's called *The Happy Face Theory with Shaman Sense.*

Lha Healing

The ancient experts of Lha healing are called *Bonpo* or shamans, and the practice is called *Bon.* They are the original medicine men and herbal healers of the new, modern Tibetan medicine.

Earlier I said that there are rituals performed by shamans who also possess all of the energy and vision possible, such as being able to heal in the presence of the person and healing at a distance, visions of past, present, and future lives, and so on. Only such shamans have the gift and permission to intervene and perform secret practices—for example, recuperating the Lha.

Some of those symptoms are brought about by either magic or trauma, such as shock due to an accident or an emotional shock such as divorce or the loss of a loved one; or by drug addiction or from prescribed antidepressants, or as a result of anesthesia used for surgical procedures. Specific symptoms include mental depression and loss of interest in things and life in general. As time passes one feels more and more afraid—afraid perhaps to be with throngs of people or having difficulty looking someone in the eye. Instead, the person stares strangely at people in kind of a side glance fashion, which some might perceive as a distrustful glare. It's difficult for such a person to accept other people. The more time that passes, the more the Lha is lost, the more their desire of isolation increases, and the more they seek darkness or hide in corners, as is often the case with schizophrenia. This creates a disturbance in the wind humor, and the individual loses radiance in the skin, becomes dehydrated, and acquires a bluish color.

A traditional physician will find nothing wrong either in pathological symptoms or causes. No allopathic tests or exams will reveal anything serious or grave. In fact, the doctor could give the person medicine that might even have some temporary effect, but it will not improve the person's health. The symptoms will reappear, like a revolving door. The risk is that an Occidental doctor will diagnose this as depression or schizophrenia and give the patient some sort of psychopharmaceutical medication or tranquilizers. This medication will give the patient a false sense of tranquility because of the sedation, not because the patient is being healed.

In this case, the only way to relieve the symptoms is to have a ritual performed by a shaman to recuperate the Lha, which has either separated from the physical body or had its connection to the body interrupted. When the Lha is completely separated, it's very dangerous because the patient cannot live very long. Premature death often results. They say people live a maximum of three years, and some say one year for the Lha completely robbed by evil spells or spirits. The enigma here is that when the Lha is distanced from the body, it does not always display chronic illness. However, our immune system is definitely at risk and vulnerable in these cases.

Evil Spirits

Let's now describe the evil spirits. These evil spirits are always on the prowl. They don't eat material food, but the food that nurtures their body is an energetic food. The spirits keep the Lha for a long time. If we do not find someone to recuperate the Lha or return it to accompany the physical body, it will be destroyed permanently.

There are two kings of the spirits that have many servants which go around the world to capture the Lha. These spirits rob the Lha via many methods of subterfuge. For example, sleeping in a forest, alone, near a lake you might find it a spot of easy prey for one of these spirits. Other types of spirits don't rob the Lha but simply absorb our energy, a little at a time.

There are also spirit possessions on a very negative and higher realm; they can take control of our will and we become slaves to their every desire until they finally bring us to the headquarters of the chief or king. These live inside of us and not only are diagnosed by the shaman's naked eye, but can be confirmed by a complicated but interesting type of urinalysis, based on its color and elements and divided into nine different houses (somewhat like that of what we know as astrological houses). Many levels and types of spirits and spirit disturbances are present—for example, those provoked by witchcraft, those of a high realm that disturb our protector spirits, and those connected to the humors. Otherwise positive spirits are provoked by our particular defilements; those that stalk in the darkness of the night; those that are provoked by or create mental or spiritual imbalance in the household or entire family; those of the field or land which adversely influence the economic resources of the family by blocking the crops or animal growth and health; those evolving around ancestral or karmic influences; those aroused by our negative actions; those related to our extreme or morose attachment to our children; those that kill animals; those that kidnap or damage or steal the Aura of man, and so on. Each of these provokes corresponding organic illnesses as well as psychological and material difficulties.

Black Magic

The other type of Lha damaging is that of black magic.[22] The black magician works on the Lha to send the negative influence toward someone, using concentration and various rituals.

This occultism interrupts the energetic connection of our birth, that which gives us stabilized form. We are basically connected and attached from three parts[23] of our physical body to our very subtle Lha toward the heavens, and this is the connection that the magician disconnects or cuts, thereby damaging the Lha of the victim.

Many types of rituals are available to protect and recover the loss of a victim's Lha, thereby recapturing its health. Another type of reality, however, cannot be saved. That is the reality of premature death as in the case of having performed or ordered someone to perform black magic on another, and that is *Sce* and *Gni*, which refer to one's personal enemy. This Gni is our mind, our conscious. When our real conscious leaves our body at the moment of death, the Lha accompanies it, reflecting this mind, until it gradually evaporates.

The Lha that is formed with us follows us in this life, thinking as we do, absorbing our sensations and all of our characteristics. At the moment of death, Lha is so strongly impregnated by our personality that it no longer possesses a real mind, and it can continue to move in place of us. This is the case of places that are infested with spirits. These are not spirits per se, but the Lha of a once-living person. If this Lha does not leave or go away with the deceased, it can actually possess someone else. It can go around normally, just as though it was that deceased person, even displaying the same character traits.

The other type of spirit invasion is that which a spirit does not possess another but is having difficulty leaving the Earth. In this case there is another type of ritual that helps the Lha of the dead or dying person to transmigrate. This ceremony is a *torma*, and it's very sweet and symbolic. In fact, it's a ceremony that often gives comfort to the surviving family. Torma releases the attachments to Earth, and then the spirit Lha goes away definitively. This restlessness and inability to move into Nirvana happens because the deceased person was either fearful of dying and wants to hold on, or a living loved one does not let him go, or in the case of sudden or unprepared death a person has some unfinished business, or the loved one has left something undone between themselves and the deceased. This situation can exist when anyone has not died at peace with oneself or the world. The job of the shaman is also to check out and assist in communications between the living and deceased parties. (Not by a medium, but only a shaman, as it's unethical to contact the dead other than to perform a shaman torma.) Such communications are done only in the case of purifying and settling the unrequited mourning period and allowing both to move on. Then the assisted departure ceremony follows immediately. Extreme Unction, the Catholic sacrament of applying the Last Rites, is an offshoot of the more complex Celtic Witch Ritual.

I feel it necessary to hammer home this idea on the subject. Since so many people are disturbing the dead and their loved ones, I need to explain further with hopes of getting my point across. We seem to be in an era when the trend is to contact a deceased soul through mediums. Uncategorically, it's not only unhealthy, unnatural, and unethical but also forbidden in the spiritual spirit world to contact any of these souls. We cannot evoke them, but if they are roaming around this plane, we may communicate with them in or out of the presence of their loved one to discover their problem. Sometimes this conversation takes one contact, and sometimes as many as five or six contacts because we must justify and satisfy their needs. If this contact is done for purely commercial or egotistical reasons or entirely at random, it can bring a great deal of harm to the medium, the requestor of the contact, and the soul contacted. The risks are death or illness to the living, negative possession, and opening channels of negativity to flow around aimlessly to the unsuspecting. On the purely psychological level, if a living person insists on continuous contact, the soul cannot rest in peace. We must always confront and learn to accept the eventual death of those around us. Otherwise we develop morbid psychoses that will bring us to the point of separating from our LHA.

Sce instead is a spirit killer, sent by the king of the spirits, which has its own mind and is the hunter that follows us for all our physical life. Gni is our mind. Sce is our inevitable death.

According to Tibetan philosophy we have what is called the "Mara of Death"—the death that no one can deny. It's inherent in our existence. No one is free from this possibility; not even Buddha can cancel its inevitability. Sce is a spirit that roams around because we must die; we can, through rituals, protect this life or extend the moment of death, but we cannot flee from it because we are impermanent. The master of death is Mara, and no one can escape him, if it's his or her time.

Case History

USA. Female, seventy-eight years old. In a nursing home. Removed and put in hospital for pneumonia. (Many operations were performed on her prior to her being placed in the nursing home.) At the hospital, the doctor diagnosed imminent death with six weeks maximum. Moved to Hospice. *Problem:* Mara of Death roaming around her environments waiting for others who are to die. Lots of spirits of Civil War soldiers on the original land of nursing home. *Esoteric diagnosis:* Mara of Death closer to a Shey spirit absorbing and separating her Aura. *Procedure:* Replace the Aura. *Second procedure:* Replenish her lost enzymes in the Aura. *Results:* Three weeks later, in hospice, and they are discharging because they say she is stable.

Summary

The Aura body, Lha, and the life force, Tse, can both be lost due to shock (such as from strong anxiety, pain, stress, drugs, or stolen by spirits). In such a case, the person gets unexpectedly and suddenly ill and dies unless the Lha can be recovered. The physical vitality (Srog) cannot be stolen, only interrupted due to loss or damage to the Tse or Lha.

The shaman explanation of death is that an assassin (Shey) spirit comes and cuts our auric body and then eats it, kind of like the Grim Reaper of the West that cuts off life with a sickle as though it's harvesting grain. Our protectors try to keep the Shey spirits away, but finally they always come and eat our auric body. The Lha can be separated from the physical body. Often, when a person has just died, people avoid the house for a while in the event that some assassin spirits may be around. In this case, the spirits do not hesitate to kill any Aura they come across.

The very subtle Lha is at the heart; only a shaman has the sight to perceive it. The gross Lha radiates out from that. This is what clairvoyant faith healers describe when we talk about the Aura.

The Srog Lha does not go with us from life to life. We receive a new one each time we reincarnate. However, when we die, sometimes when our consciousness goes onto the next life, our Lha remains behind for a while in the world. In fact, all ancient religions believe that neither a cremation nor organ removal should be performed before thirty-six hours of the official expiration. Even until modern times, for example, the Jewish religion does not bury or cremate their deceased brethren for at least thirty-six hours. There are multiple accounts of people seeing a detached auric double and mistaking it for the person's ghost, as it can appear and talk to mediums. A person who is really reborn as a spirit has a "spirit body," not an auric body. Spirits can only harm our auric body, not our gross body. Sorcerers and magicians with strong psychic powers can use their own auric body to attack the Auras of others. This is why we need different methods of auric protection.

The black magic operator can use many physical items to harm the Lha and Tse, such as hair and personal clothing, photos, and so on. I know of a case in which the companion of an unsuspecting man took a black statue to a black magician, who put a certain powder in the statue. While the husband was asleep, she pronounced certain chants that the magician gave her. The purpose was to control and destroy his love life and to make him shyer and more timid than normal with women—to forget any other woman past, present, or future, except his companion, whether alive or not. This case is sad because the selfishness and evil are multifold. These actions will make the husband die prematurely, because it's black magic and all black magic of this level eventually kills the person. Second, she knew that she had little time to live herself because of a critical illness that she did not tell him about—a selfish act. Third, there was a little baby in the middle of this. If both adults die, the baby will be parentless. According to dharma, the person who participates in these negative actions will receive unsuspecting recourse either in this life or in the next. Remember, "What goes around comes around." Or as they say in India, "We give out what we get back."

Here we have a very complicated case, because the victim—basically a good soul with a very good heart and sense of responsibility—while weakened by life's circumstances and multiple black magic attacks, is very controlled and dominated by his partner. Already having a timid personality, this situation created more mental confusion and anger inside him. This began to be manifested in violence, because his Lha was separated by all of these traumas, which had deleterious effects on his vital energy, leaving him even less able to fight back.

Wind symptoms created dizziness, a lot of yawning, bad digestion, and a nervous stomach (an exacerbation of the symptoms he previously suffered due to his humor imbalances from years of black magic, mental abuse, and lack of motherly affection). In this case, it was necessary after such multiplicity of negativity to evaluate the new situation.

The man should ask permission from a higher power to heal his Lha and examine if a karmic lesson was learned, and to negate the psychic power of this statue. Then he should observe his condition astrologically,[24] including examining the series of other emotional childhood problems that was often released by spurts of misdirected pugilism, and attempt to bring back his Lha. Astrologically, they call this "feeling his ascendant," or his basic character that as an adult he kept under control.

Because of the black witchcraft rituals against him, he is regressing without being aware of why or how. When a person loses one's Lha due to witchcraft, he or she regresses always to a state of infancy or youth, basically demonstrating the exaggerated negative form of their character. Tibetan astrologers refer to it as an imbalance of one of the elements of wood, metal, fire, water, or earth. I offer you this understanding, so that if you should encounter situations of this sort you might be able to demonstrate more self-control, if perhaps it's you that is damaged; and you might be able to demonstrate comprehension, tolerance, and patience toward another who might have been a victim of such destruction. When the Lha has been separated, the physical and mental damages take some time to completely calm down and disappear, and a single action of removing negativity or replacing the Lha is not sufficient for a total healing. The shaman must analyze other damage that has taken place as a result of the energetic situation, go back in, and heal that as well. In other words, removing the negativity alone is not sufficient, and healing is a long process. Don't expect to rebuild Rome in a day; patience and understanding are the key words in these cases.

A participating victim always makes the shaman's labor a little easier. It's helpful to have a willing individual or an intermediary who is aware of the problem and the need to address it, but it's not always necessary. It's just that the shaman's work is more difficult and takes longer to see its immediate effect. You will notice little glimpses of improvements, slowly; again, time depends on the base character of the person and the particular astrological aspects of the geographic and global aspects of the time.

In this case and in many others we can influence our Lha positively by various physical actions (like cold showers), mantras, and visualizations. Also, discovering the lessons one is supposed to learn from all of this offers another karmic lesson of this life. As in the above case, the karmic lessons are that the victim of the black magic must learn what it's like to be really loved, a love of compassion and respect. He should learn to find the courage to approach the person or woman who is complete spiritually and with good intentions in life who can give him sincere, unconditional love. He is also to learn to take better control of his life and not let others dominate him, to find company that is more synergetic with his virtues and more supportive of his needs. This is only a start at finding peace and equilibrium. All this must be performed—he must develop more courage, relinquish his fears and doubts about himself, and display more will and determination. This lesson is being carried over from another life, and he had better learn it now. Otherwise, he will continue to find himself in various themes of the same scenarios until he decides to complete this particular karma. This spiritual follow-up consultation is the ideal situation for the healing shaman, because it's possible to help the person to understand karmically the lesson he is to learn, and then to rectify the problem. In the end we are able to put into the hands of the afflicted an indispensable tool of self-healing.

If we know someone who has lost his or her Lha, the only thing we can do is to bring them to a positive, spiritual shaman. The shaman then recalls the life essence by performing certain rituals, sometimes even paying a ransom for the Lha, sometimes buying animals destined for slaughter and releasing them, and so on. Recuperating the Lha is not sufficient. We have to go in and restructure the person from the detrimental effects on all three levels, and then return for total protection against further damage or ill effects.

In all cases, if our auric energy is strong, our risks are slim to none that any of these negativities, demonic or otherwise, can reenter and control us. In fact, often I see these critters, the negativity, looming around the outer shell of an Aura waiting for a moment of weakness, perhaps a minor, otherwise insignificant illness such as a long-term virus. And even then, the spirits cannot do as much harm to the strong as to the weak. In the case of a stronger character, the entities can annoy and block or delay our destiny.

Perhaps you have a feeling of occasional nervousness and anxiety, or feel that for every ten steps in life you take it's almost as though something or someone is pulling you backward eight steps. A feeling of incompleteness emerges, and progress is thwarted. For these reasons, we need different methods of auric protection.

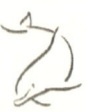

Chapter 17

Self-Healing and Self-Actualization
Meditations for Clearing Negativity and Completing Karma

First, regarding negativity or protection from negativity:

1. It's negative in itself to discuss or analyze who placed this negativity on us. Instead, dwell on the spiritual and karmic causes inside of us.
2. Meditate for protection from further harm.
3. Meditate on clearing your faith blocks. We have a need to believe in *the* superior being, whether you believe it's us or something else. It really doesn't matter. Human beings by their very nature need faith to exist. Which belief system we follow depends on how we were raised or what we brought with us from another life and how we visualize it and retrieve it.
4. Self-analyze. What were we supposed to learn from this continuous negativity placed upon us? Ask Aura, "Why am I attracting this? Is there something I'm supposed to learn? Is there some behavior of my life that I must alter or change?"
5. Seek the resolution: "What am I doing or not doing that can end this continuous assault that I permit?'Acknowledgment: "Yes, I recognize that I allow this to happen and I can end it through my karmic growth via meditation, prayer, and introspection."

6. Implement intelligent remorse: Reflect on the one action that you performed the day before that you would like to change because it might have been an action that hurt someone or something via word, thought, or deed, or which illustrated lack of compassion. This could have been as simple as prejudging someone. Next, make a promise, without guilt, for the next twenty-four hours to not have such thoughts, words, or negative deeds.
7. Be grateful. Reflect on something that someone did for you within the last few days that was nice. Thank that person in this meditation and reflect on the feeling of joy that it gave you.
8. Wake up every morning with a positive purpose, a positive motivation, or raison d'être. A sense of purpose seems to encourage a more positive outlook toward our sufferings. What we know, we can combat.
9. Unravel your natural gifts and talents and eventually seek to be working or perhaps even earning our living from that for which we are naturally adapted. Don't work only because you want money or because you are afraid of being without money. Money comes as a byproduct of living in peace and harmony and having a career or profession that one was born to do, and second, that gives us gratification. Then we will even have more control on our use of time and be able to better harmonious all aspects of our life—social, career, spiritual, hobbies, pleasures, pastimes, and so on. We can have it all.
10. We can consider going back to the same shaman to help us to regress to find out what these past lives' weaknesses are, while also finding out our past-life strengths, talents, and wisdom to try to enhance or reawaken them (whatever the case might be) in your current life. Then incorporate them into a meditation and actually communicate with your Aura. You can ask your Aura out loud to give you what you are lacking. You can also ask your Aura to reinforce your strengths for this life and those that you carry forward from previous consciousnesses (lives).
11. Last but not least, embody the will and determination to evolve. Grow without fear and with faith in God or

in something or someone. The intrinsic nature of all human beings is to have a strong need for faith. It's the never-ending key to healing, without which it is difficult to survive and be peaceful. We often suffer from fear of the unknown because of a mistaken definition of the word "change." There is even a distorted interpretation of the proverb, "We know what we have, but we don't know what we will get." Change is not a negative word; with God's help and good, clear judgment, we make the correct choices and overcome.

Case History

Male, thirty-two years old. The medics found no pathological reasons for his suddenly having lost his sight. Energetically examined, however, the lack of faith was the reason. He started a few years prior to his loss of sight to rebel against his religious practices and beliefs. It was previously his heartfelt desire to faithfully attend church. During that period of time he also prayed and lit candles in church every time he entered one. I suggested to him the simple cure of going to three churches and lighting three candles for thirty days. He looked at me with skepticism and dismay because he had expected an energetic healing ceremony since he had been recommended to me as an energetic healer. He was a little disillusioned and unwilling to follow the recommendation because of a preconceived notion that I would perform a healing. When I suggested a do-it-yourself proactive exercise, he was not ready to take the responsibility for his own healing. With some considerable coaxing I was able to convince him. He did so, and three and one half months later without alternative or official medicine, he miraculously regained his sight—in essence, excuse the double entendre, he saw the light. This was a clear-cut case of how humans need to believe and not rebel against their very nature.

All of the steps outlined at the beginning of this chapter can reinforce and strengthen our Lha for the entire day, even if we only have time that day to wake up with a positive purpose. That is sufficient to eventually build a reinforced security wall around us.

Whatever we want to do in life—whether we want a successful career, a good life materially, or we want to develop our pure crystal energies in order to heal others and ourselves—we need to purify and take care of the five elements: air (wind), space, water, fire, and earth. All the energies in our environment and our life are based upon these five elements. If they are polluted or blackened, then nothing works quite right in our life.

Antinegativity Meditation

If you are really pressed for time and are not very interested in learning to meditate on profound issues or for too long a period of time, you can simply perform the following, which works for general protection from negative energies:

1. Go into meditation as suggested previously. Then begin to visualize yourself and your Aura—or even just your physical being, if you cannot yet see your Aura.
2. Create the visual of a white tent.
3. Envision your body, physical and auric, living in the tent. (The Tibetans call this a Vajra Tent.) It's a house where we can sleep and perform all our daily activities peacefully without fear of negative energy. Inside this tent we experience reality as a very blissful environment. Allow your mind to relax into the experience of relative and absolute Space. If we can visualize this tent as enormous, almost like the size of a villa, we can eventually put people, such as our children, inside. If you, however, are in a particular negative state of mind, filled with lots of personal problems, don't put anyone else in this tent for the time being.

My mother taught me this and another, even simpler mental picture, as in the following story. She taught us this to accompany the use of the Crystal Fairy Scepter (visit the Auraology site to get your scepter) for us to chase away the bogeyman. She employed many such exercises, playfully and intelligently, as she was teaching us crystal therapy so we could relate to it. It really worked. All sentiments encompassed in fear as well as phobias that we deemed frightful or just plain disliked dissipated.

4. Take an actual or imaginary crystal wand and clear all the space around your physical body with this crystal.[25] Visualize the negativity being erased and cleared away. (The only problem with this step is that it does not seem to protect us from catching the bug if we don't get methodical about self-protection because of our hectic lifestyles. To remain consistent, we have to use gemstones to achieve blocking negativity, purifying and reinforcing the Aura from the damages that occur when preventing various flagellations or disease. Tools such as the Auraology Magic Fairy Scepter and the purpose healing wand help, as do the Neptune Scepter and other healing jewelry, both for individuals and energy healers.)

5. Envision a white light that is bathing you and protecting you in all its glory. This takes only seconds to do and can be accomplished while walking down the street or riding in the car to work.

Tibetan Feng Shui.
Tantra Meditation Position
Meditation can be improved sitting in the center of these directions

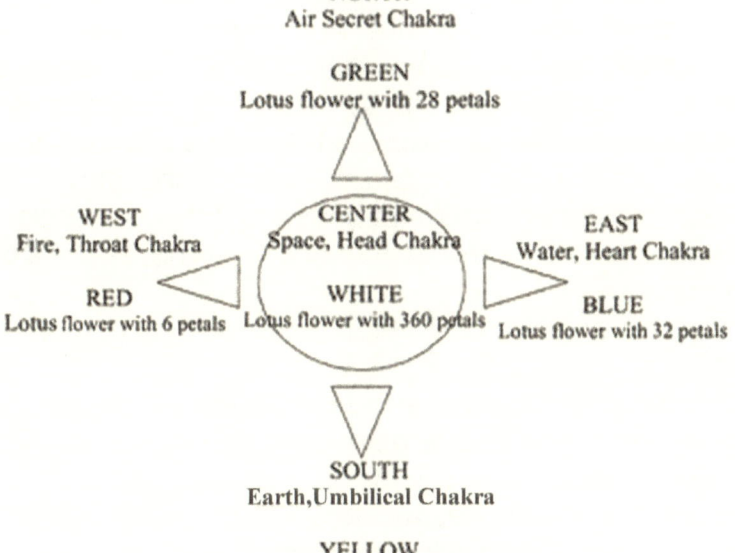

NORTH
Air Secret Chakra

GREEN
Lotus flower with 28 petals

WEST
Fire, Throat Chakra

CENTER
Space, Head Chakra

EAST
Water, Heart Chakra

RED
Lotus flower with 6 petals

WHITE
Lotus flower with 360 petals

BLUE
Lotus flower with 32 petals

SOUTH
Earth,Umbilical Chakra

YELLOW
Lotus flower with 64 petals

Another Simple Protective Shield Meditation

1. Visualize your inner auric body armor like a membrane of golden, pure crystal light between our flesh and skin, so that none of our inner energy can leak out, and no dark or harmful energy can enter or injure our crystal-light body. By wearing the pure crystal body armor, we can connect through our umbilical channel (the center channel) with our inner Shambhala. Wearing this crystal-light body armor allows us to enter into any situation and always be relaxed, knowing that we are protected. This and the other self-healing meditations presented here protect you from psychic attacks; you will see a clear and healthy complexion and at the same time prolong your life.

Other, More Involved Meditations

Many varieties of meditations with their corresponding mantras work on every aspect of our being, physical and spiritual. Some such meditations are the transformation of the five elements and consciousness within our own body and mind and then offering this pure energy to the holy beings; meditation on the empty body (Srong Ra); meditation on strengthening the Tse (life force); meditation (done by physicians and energy healers) to purify the body, mind, and spirit, so as not to absorb illnesses from patients and not to infect the patients with whatever illnesses the healer might have; meditations to purify our words, thoughts, deeds, and actions, both gross and subtle; meditations to purify the inner and outer environment based on lotus meditations; and meditations to reinforce the astrological weaknesses of a person. The list goes on.

There are procedures in Tibetan Tantra called *initiations*. These are meditations and blessings brought to you through qualified monks to present you with various understandings, realizations, and teachings. When one is appropriately initiated in this realm via the designated monk (lama), that person can then practice with success the mantras associated with the initiation and impart them onto others. These initiations have brief and long formats. Obviously, the long form is more likely to be performed only in the Oriental environment because of the depth of the philosophy and because the length of these ceremonies is too difficult for the Western mind to grasp because of cultural differences. For example, the normal time period for a formal Vajrayogini Initiation is three months, while the short form is a week. Even lately I've heard of such an initiation that is even shorter, a half-day in length. However, if you hear of certain initiations being given, rest assured that the lamas who have been given the power for that particular teaching will be dynamite. Those who have been given the responsibility or approval to impart it have sufficiently and deeply studied the particular philosophy.

Certain oaths/initiations of the medicine Buddha, for example, must be taken by Tibetan physicians; those of Vajrayogini are good for people who work in the mental healing arts. Many more examples are available. All are sufficiently complex and long.

I pass on to you now a very important mantra that everyone can say for protection against further negativity, once it has been removed from you. It's more appropriately stated as transformed from negative to positive. This negativity includes and is not limited to your own negativity. While visualizing that light in the space between the hair and the flesh of our body, repeat these words:

OM MUNI MUNI MAHA MUNI SHAKYAMUNIE SOHA

The words mean as follows:

Om: Mental calm and happiness.

Muni: The determination to abandon suffering.

Muni: Represents the mind that wishes to help all other sentient beings.

Maha Muni: Represents the correct vision of reality. The perception that all phenomena are by nature empty, free from any existing conformity.

Shakyamunie: Represents the secret Tantric passageway or path. It's the most rapid. Missions of Buddhas are in the Buddhist religion, but the Shakyamunie Buddha is the only one that transmits the Tantric teachings.

Soha: I pray to you, supplicate you, to please concede to me these realizations.

This mantra has its origin in the Buddha Shakyamunie. All divinities have their origins in Buddha Shakyamunie for the Shambhala of Kalachakra, the Wheel of Wisdom.

*   *   *

Here's another mantra, a method for transforming our world into a pure and simple land. Say three times,

HUM AH OM

Air: *Hum* (Inhale) Illuminates all the impurities of color, smell, and potential (white).

Fire: *Ah* (Hold your breath) Transforms them into nectar (red).

Water: *Om* (Exhale) Multiplies all of the above and allows them to increase (blue).

Why Is a Mantra Important?

In all religions, words, chants, and mantras are a vibration level that work even if we are not of that religious belief. Mantras have an effect on us regardless, because they work on the sound energy level and not the intellectual level. Among Christian mantras are the Alleluia, the Kyrie, the Doxology, and so on. They are kinds of friends most near to us; they are stable, always helping us and always being good companions. I knew that when I learned Gregorian chant and sang in church, and to this day each time I chant them, I feel younger, spiritually rejuvenated, uplifted, and purified. So it's no coincidence that all religions use chants. I also tested these Tibetan chants along with the Kyrie and many others on the Karnak Sensor of Luciano Muti. He validated that the intended purification of the recited mantras coincided with the registration on the graphic impulses or frequencies of the brain schematic to give the particular healing energy that the ancients said it would impose. It works not only because the computer readouts confirmed it but also because I've witnessed the firsthand healing effects. Another phenomenon of Tibetan medicine in relationship to mantras is that only monks in prayer are permitted to handle the pills in the pharmacology laboratory. Many, in this case, wonder if these mantra vibrations make the medicines so potent. In addition, "precious pills,"[26] as they are called, are taken under certain phases of the moon for psychological disorders and are assigned accompanying mantras that are recommended to be recited by the patient when ingesting these pills. We derive benefits from the mantras even if we mispronounce them, and even without understanding their intended final effect. All these help us to realize illumination and find the strength and faith to continue onward in our quest. Try them.

Past and Present Life Reflections—Karmic Regression

After negativity has been transformed and you have been performing protective meditations, think about your next phase: discovering the why and what you must learn from this. Begin to ask the shaman to help you to discover your past lives. Orthodox Buddhist doctrine says don't even think about the reasons and the lessons. It just is. I believe there is a happy medium between the two . . . . You don't obsess over it, but you can be aware of the necessity of a particular karma for a particular incident.

Case in point: When I was a violent crime victim I felt that my healing was directly related to discovering and eliminating the karmic reasons for what had happened. There were many, and I will share one with you. According to astrologically analysis, the two individuals who were in my house and left me for dead had been in my most previous past life. They were border guards and both males. I was trying to cross a European border to bring food and money to a psychiatrist that was performing important research in his center for schizophrenia. In this lifetime the perpetrators were male and female. The individuals wanted food from me; I decided to give them money and not the food as food was at a high premium for those in the center to survive. The guards were not happy. I wanted to do it my way. I had to complete that cycle. Maybe I did and maybe I did not at the time of the attack. But perhaps I did when I danced off to Italy like Mary Poppins to fulfill a mission. Only then did I learn what it means to change your style of doing things as it's done somewhere else. Of course, I mean that this is done without exaggerating who you are or compromising your morals, but adapting and being aware.

Think about and ask yourself the following:

1. What was/were the most important lesson(s) I learned in that and this life?
2. What do I like the most about the person I was in that life and who I am in this life?
3. What do I dislike most about the person I was in that and this life?
4. What negative influences from that and this life (situations, events, character traits, etc.) are still affecting who and what I am in this life?
5. What positive influences from that and this life—such as situations, events, character traits, and talents—are still affecting me in this lifetime?
6. Are any of the individuals I know in my current life people I knew in that life, and how has our past-life relationship affected our current circumstances?

Remember that the goal of this exercise is to unearth answers to questions that will help you get out of your messes now. For example, if you come to the realization that in a past life you were a leader, but in your present life you are now a shy person or unable even to manage simple situations effectively, you should use the information you have uncovered to help you realize that leadership qualities still reside latently within you. Then you simply ask your Aura to reawaken the bravery, assertiveness, and ability to manage complex situations that you possessed in a previous life—for example, as a general of the army of ancient Rome.

You can even reawaken and enhance past and present life talents and wisdom in the current life. For example, I would like to learn to accept the compassion I possess and demonstrate toward others today as when I was a Buddhist monk in Tibet in order to enhance my current ability to love and to be generous with others without the fear of being hurt by the person that I befriend. You can do the same with past and present life traumas, pains, and negative patterns that you would like to heal or overcome in this life.

One sweet-smelling summer day on the beach at 6 a.m., I guided a man into a karmic regression meditation. I had read in his Aura during the first visit that he was suffering from lack of courage to confront his mother and lack of courage to confront certain types of conflicts. He also suffered from colon spasms, which is a classic symptom according to Tibetan medicine for his emotional and psychological difficulties. He mostly responded to people's requests with a sense of guilt. Having suggested to him that he was a likely candidate for looking into these lives for the resolution, we did so. We voyaged together into this lifetime and saw he was a officer in command of foot soldiers who was betrayed by one of his underlings, who purposely gave the soldiers incorrect orders. He went out to assist the foot soldiers in danger, could not reach them because his horse reared up from fear, and the officer fell. His traitor pierced his stomach with a sword. He died, with a sense of guilt and incompetency as a leader. This is the cause of his intestinal problems in this lifetime: his hesitancy to take on leadership roles of importance. We are still working on these problems, but he has circumvented the need for years of psychotherapy just in the first sitting by identifying the real problem and from whence it came. That is 50 percent of the battle. In addition, from the Tibetan point of view, these emotions give just those physical disorders—not to mention the coincidence that he was stabbed in the stomach and suffers from gastrointestinal problems.

Take each set of suggestions and then gradually ask yourself all of these questions, in meditation or at a time when you have no distractions and no one else is around you. Visualize these situations. Visualize yourself in the positive, not the negative. Say to yourself, *I am courageous. I deserve to be loved.* And feel inside of yourself and outside of you a person who will give you love.

I suggest keeping a journal on all of this.

A negative occurrence in this life does not mean that you were a bad person in a previous life. If someone robbed me, that doesn't necessarily mean I was previously a thief. It could simply mean I needed to acquire more humility or that I placed too much emphasis on material worth. That you are rich today doesn't mean that you were a princess in a previous life.

By the way, don't get illusions of grandeur. Most of us curiously begin to trace former lives with the conscious or unconscious idea that we were only of the elite in previous lives. Not always true; be careful not to project what you want to see or believe. Karma does not work like that. Things are much simpler. For example, as a young, newly divorced woman in the United States, I realized that every man in my life, whether romantic or in family relationships, took precedence over my own professional and personal goals. When I say "took precedence," it was me not them who initiated these time-consuming distractions. In fact, often if the favors were not returned or men did not thank me, my feelings were hurt. I was expecting something in return, unconsciously. This is called "giving with strings"—"giving," because you consciously or unconsciously want something in return. In this case we demonstrate a lack of humility, anticipating that we can cure everybody—the "all things to all people" syndrome—or in the case of female evolutionary difficulties, American psychiatrists call this the *Superwoman Syndrome*. Tibetans call it *attachment*.

I started analyzing my upbringing and concluded that it was exactly the opposite of how I was raised, but I was the one allowing this to happen. My father was not a chauvinist, did not make demands on me, and in fact his big dream was always to have me in business with him. Strange, because I have two brothers, and usually for an Italian American man the big dream was to be in business with his sons, not his daughter. Okay, looking at this, I gave my present life ten points. No root to the problem here. So how come I keep making the same stupid mistakes?

My brother had a need for me to always be there, putting my own career development on hold. My ex-husband had illusions of being a big industrialist and financier, so I began to put my career on hold and obtain the financial licenses needed to start a stock brokerage firm—putting my studies aside, which at the time was to be medicine. After my divorce, a new fiancé entered, and again, the same pattern. I put my career on hold in deference to his needs. At this point I said, *enough*. Time to find out why.

I already knew what career and professional path I was to be taking that was consistent with my natural capabilities of being a psychological and anatomical healer. I would put them aside for the needs (often unexpressed) of that man in my life. I was on a merry-go-round, and I finally chose to put on the brakes. But I did not understand why I was doing it. I decided to regress into past lives.

The first series of lives I saw were that of what seemed to be a Spanish peasant woman working in the fields, sheathing grain. I heard and saw her weeping for the wrongdoings of her nine sons. The scene took me into the village where she lived. I discovered that all of her nine sons were either killed or in jail for some sort of delinquency or another. In essence, they were all failures. I felt her sense of guilt. She felt it was all her fault. Then I saw her death. She died sobbing with guilt.

Well, that did it. As a child, without provocation, just the slightest offense perpetrated on me or a certain look from my mother threw me into automatic sobbing. My brother gave me the nickname "Crocodile Tears." Then I understood clearly why I felt it necessary to be responsible for all the male creatures in my life. I was trying to make up for what I did not do well previously.

We know that is objectively absurd. At that moment, having been aware of the problem was 80 percent of the solution. But this was not sufficient to eliminate the emotional difficulty.

I began a simple exercise. Every morning, I looked myself in the mirror and said, *I love you, Patricia.* I then started chanting, "No." This was a word I had difficulty uttering when someone had a perceived need, but you can and must do what God wants of you. When I had sufficient time I began meditating, visualizing me no longer as the personal slave of the men in my life and carrying through with what God asked of me for Him.

At that precise time entered a new fiancé. That was evolved and helped me to develop just that capacity, to take time to develop that which I needed, yet to develop academically and career-wise to fulfill my prewritten destiny, because he was nonchauvinistic and very supportive of my career and emotional development. Now I know how to balance, both with a healthy attitude, relaxed and without guilt, and without expectations from the other person. Now it takes a lot more than a slight offense to drive me into tears.

I leave this otherwise very complicated exploration with another word of warning. The only good reason for questioning your past lives is in order to improve your present situation, not for frivolous motives. Look and see what relationship these previous lives have with this life, and then move forward by applying this learning lesson. Karmic regression is not a parlor game; it's instead an effective tool that, when repeated, can help you to stop bungling up your life. We can only heal what we understand.

What to Do after a Tibetan Shaman Has Transformed Negativity

The other thing we should do on a physical level is to change a few of our habits particularly for thirty days after a shaman has transformed the negativity or restored your Lha.

1. Take only cold showers. Better yet, bathe in a natural spring. Visualize that all-negative energies and auric pollution are washed away. These showers are beneficial for strengthening the Aura. They help reduce tiredness and increase vitality, sexual energy, and blood circulation. Phlegmatic people should avoid this advice, as it will increase their psychophysical imbalance.
2. If you are not allergic to cow's milk, drink fresh milk with honey (otherwise, goat's milk).
3. Do not cook with oil. Use either nothing or purified butter such as ghee butter for cooking.
4. Drink meat broth daily, preferably beef or game. By all means, do not use pork or chicken. This increases ignorance and attachment.
5. Wear gold, especially over your heart, which as you recall is the seat of our auric body.

According to your individual dietary or health needs, for at least one month eliminate all foods with the exception of beef or game, yogurt and honey. This will definitely strengthen your Aura and very subtle illusory body. If you are a vegan or vegetarian you can substitute with vegetable/barley miso soup; almond spread, cocoanut oils but never use olive oil for cooking it is only a condiment after you have steamed the veggies. You can take a tablespoon of crude extra virgin olive oil before retiring to help your digestion.

In all cases avoid meat from animals that have been saturated with steroids and hormones. One of our body's waste products, if you recall from earlier on in the book, is a sexual hormone.

Taking in artificial hormones through our diet via our food or contraceptive pills may well damage the protective shield of our Aura and leave us with a defenseless immune system. I once read a medical science research paper from the National Institute of Health indicating that women who have taken birth control pills are more susceptible to AIDS as compared to women who have never taken birth control pills. (This, by the way, creates a false pregnancy in the body in order to further prevent pregnancy.)

Addendum

We have spoken about self-healing through the reading of the Aura. I have also explained the principles of the Tibetan Tantra with the hopes that you might begin to embark on a new philosophical approach to life. It's a universal dogma that will whet your appetite and stimulate the desire for an alternative lifestyle, one that will convert your pessimistic comportment (to which we all sooner or later fall prey) into a positive and more beneficial approach to life management. The perpetual state of resignation, letting the events of life control us instead of our controlling those events, brings us continuous insurmountable sufferings.

Unfortunately, no pills can supplant this long and arduous task. Hard work, commitment, and putting aside our ego are the only ways to embark on this road to spiritual betterment.

Winston Churchill said, "A pessimist is one who makes difficulties of his opportunities, and an optimist is one who makes opportunities of his difficulties." Yet if we learn to see things in the spiritual light, and comprehend that all that happens is our destiny, we can better accept and understand all the vicissitudes often encountered in life.

I'm not suggesting that life will be without bumps in the road, but through diligent preparation and comprehension we can acquire the tools and grit necessary to achieve bliss. We can have the awareness that these bumpy, uneven streets are not obstacles to our journey, but nothing more than fortunate opportunities presented to us for our eventual emergence from the of Samsara and their Milestones. The results depend entirely on us. How we decide to cope, our degree of commitment, and our indomitable spirit are directly proportional to the final results.

Will we take a laissez-faire attitude and let others control events? Will we continue to let events control us? Or will we pray and labor for reinforced determination and will? And via this spiritual approach will we thereby become the kings and queens of our destiny?

Always maintain an open mind, a consciousness that will ask, when you think or dream of something that has never happened, "Why not?" instead of "Why?" If you should experience negative attitudes, transform them into white light; this light not only extends our physical life but guarantees a high quality of life, one that permits us to enjoy good health and acute and limpid minds.

However, for those of you who already maintain the positive quality of an open mind and have embraced the Dharma Samsara, you can use these principles to benefit all of society in general.

After successfully completing the personal application and implementation of this spiritual voyage, you are prepared to perpetuate and promulgate the theories. Take your family and then your friends by the hand and put them in the Samsara vehicle. After all, this is the end goal of pure enlightenment: sharing the Word.

In all cases, however, no matter what road you choose—whether only to help yourself or to amplify this circle by teaching others—I advise you to try to conduct your life in a Dharma manner.

The Dharma Doctrine

Always keep promises. Otherwise we risk losing self-esteem and the esteem of others, therefore losing our true worth. When we decide to do something, whether on the physical, mental, or verbal level, if our mind takes a negative direction or if we embark on a negative route, we must immediately change directions. On the other hand, if you make a promise that is impossible to keep because when you made that promise you were not aware of the reasons or motivations behind the request, and you find after time that you did not have all the facts or some of the facts were hidden from you at the time, or you later realized that keeping the promise would produce harm to yourself or others, then you must and can without second thought change directions and break that promise. However, if, for example, we are performing an act that is positive, such as at work or the simplest promise to a child to take her for ice cream, even if we are tired and we want to abandon this accord we must continue and not turn back on our word.

Therefore, before you agree to something, think it through well. Make sure you have all the information at hand and have thought out the consequences prior to making a commitment. And once you have started, you must go the whole nine yards and complete the journey.

Advice for Developing a Dharma-Positive Attitude

Don't listen to negative social information, such as gossip and sensationalistic news headlines. Look for the truth and the positive aspects in the daily bombardment of unfiltered information.

The Dharma Samsara is the base fundamental of a happy life. The Tantra is not teaching anything beyond our reach or beyond our comprehension, because all human beings deep down desire peace, joy, and good health. This desire sometimes creates a strong related desire, however, for something. If the goal of this something is a positive attitude or freedom from suffering, we will succeed using the principles and practices I've shared with you in these pages. They are attainable by everyone in their simplest forms. Although they might sound unconventional to you at first, try to put them on and wear them for a while. You might find that you like them.

This book has also illustrated many possibilities regarding paranormal phenomena and your personal development. This is only the tip of the iceberg.

Never employ these powers or the powers of others such as black magicians to harm people; otherwise, your karma and perplexities will deepen and not clarify. And you always get back what you give out.

All of the answers to all of the questions and doubts are inside of you, and only you can unravel them, with a little nudge and a guide from a shaman. When you are filled with too many questions, you are not yet listening to the responses inside of you. When you begin to listen, and together we can get there, you will feel the force and power move you like a cannon shot. When you get this feeling of mind expansion—and you will—in little leaps at a time, you are then able to recognize your improved evolutionary state and eventually become a globetrotter of the universal spiritual, feeling, and miraculous world.

Use karmic regression prudently. The only good reason for finding out about your past and present lives is to grow and benefit from what you learn. You will not glean this result if you allow ego enlargement to become a factor in compiling your notebook. Be discerning, and remember that your interest in any one of your previous or present personalities should always be commensurate with what that incarnation has to teach you about your life in the here and now.

Remember to respect the shaman. Never be so egotistical and self-centered to ask her or him questions about your life in public or without a specific appointment. That creates bad karma for you and for the shaman or other esoteric arts practitioner.

Be cautious not to fall into an egotistical trap. Never believe or think yourself to be infallible. Often the novice or the non spiritual practitioner of the esoteric arts is too ready, willing, and able to offer an opinion without having been asked. Not only is this behavior audaciously inappropriate, but it demonstrates a lack of humility. Never read someone's Aura voluntarily. If asked, only do so in a discreet time and place. Always maintain a positive outlook. Learn to be diplomatic as to how and when we inform others of what we see.

Above all, develop and seek out others who have developed a set of professional principles and ethics in guiding and transforming the energy of others. Do not frequent or become a convenient clairvoyant who does whatever is the mode of the time to profit on the weaknesses of others. (I know a young woman who accidentally killed herself in a car crash from a drunken stupor the same day a so-called psychic card reader told her that her mother was going to die. The woman client was a recovering alcoholic. After the news she went on a binge. The mother is still alive, but the girl is no longer with us.

All of us, even you, can be a mini-Shaman—a psychic surgeon pulling out all the dirt, pollution, and negativity from our bodies and minds in the form of auric mucus and letting it dissolve into absolute space. This can leave the world around us and ourselves a little bit better because we dissipated this mucus and do not allow it to stick to our hands or to anything anymore. We can do so only if we remain modest with the purest and untainted intentions, compassion, benevolence, and faith.

And last, but not least, stop defiling yourself, and . . .

Insist and resist.

And you will conquer your hidden faculties—

All of them good . . . because, after all, we are all children of God.

May the Goddesses, God, Buddha, Krishna, and Allah bless you and keep you in His/Her Protective Mantle.

I leave you only temporarily, wishing you all beauty and harmony and to be always in the "pink," and with the words of French novelist and critic Lon Bloy: "Man has places in his heart, which do not yet exist, and into them enters suffering in order that they may have existence."

You have a life to live. Now go out and live it, using the power you have inside of you!

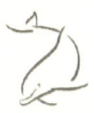

Appendix A

Other Useful Antinegativity Practices
Detoxification or Decontamination Guide

(Taken from Lama Ganchen teachings; to be hung in your meditation area)

The purpose of striving to become a mini-Yogi or to follow a dharma (spiritual path) is not only to develop mental effects, but to have a direct influence on a physical body and at a microorganism level. Therefore, in practicing this theory we transform all tainted energy into positive energy. When we become illuminated in all Wisdom, it's not only because we mentally are illuminated but also because all the energies, physical and subtle areas, are manifested into a body of wisdom.

To help you with this life's task, I have listed defilements we want to eliminate in our day-to-day lives.

Anti defilement Practices

Suggestions for the layperson (I say "layperson" because people in religious orders have an entirely more rigid set of rules):

Eliminate the following ten negative actions:

Negative Actions on the Physical Body

1. Killing animals and humans
2. Stealing (petty theft, white-collar crime included)
3. Incorrect sexual activity

Their offsetting karmic results: killing—a brief life span; stealing—rebirth into a state of poverty; incorrect sexual activity—remaining lonely and alone or having a hellish family life.

Negative Mental Actions (Thoughts)

4. Coveting goods that others have (avidity)
5. Malevolence (wishing harm to others)
6. Incorrect vision (Irrationality)

The negative result of incorrect vision is the most dangerous of the three because we lose the fundamentals of all good faith practice. The others are negative but not so damaging.

Negative Speech Actions

7. Fibbing or lying
8. Speaking uselessly (gossiping)
9. Using harsh words
10. Defamation, pitting one person against another.

The negative results are as follows: fibbing—our words lose power and no one believes us; speaking without good reason—either makes us mute or gives us difficulty in communication, such as stuttering; harsh words—our words and voice become unpleasant; defamation—friendlessness.

If we should fall, as it's human to fall, we can perform offsetting actions that will build us a kind of merit book. A Lama Ganchen, a special lama alchemist/physician/philosopher, posed the following when asked just this:

Question: What can we do when we are filled with anger?

Answer from Lama Ganchen Rinpoche: If we have money in the bank, we spend it and then we must deposit other money. The same thing happens when we are assailed by anger. If we are filled with anger for an entire day, we must on the following day accumulate Merits. (Do something nice for someone and offer it to offset the previous anger rage.) When we succeed in transforming this anger into merits (good deeds) it means that we have transformed the anger itself into energy for accumulating merits. We often experience anger, but we accumulate positive energy. Slowly this negative energy of anger weakens us, just like the deposit and withdrawal process of a bank account. We can also recite a mantra to offset enraged feelings.

Then, one day will arrive when we are tired of always being angry and our mind will gradually and slowly begin to transform.

Afterword

Practical Analysis of the ESP Qualities of Patricia Pellicciotti

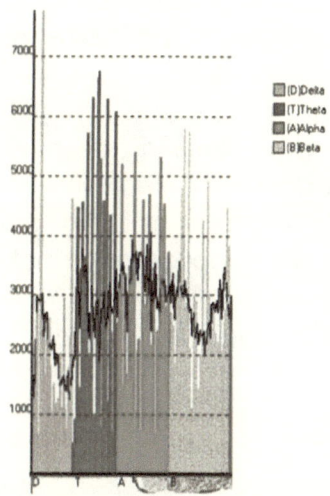

The Psychic Karnak Sensor—as large as a VHS videocassette, connected to a personal computer, with its decoded software, from a distance of one to two meters—measures the electromagnetic frequency that the human brain emits from 0.5 to 80 Hz. This device does so without the need of connecting electrodes to the head or the body of the person.

The electromagnetic frequency captured permits the analysis of the state of consciousness establishing the mental quantities such as: will, analysis—intuition, creativity, clairvoyance, and magnetism.

The Karnak Psychic Sensor displays the paranormal faculties of a healer, sensitive or prognostic, defining their degree of operative and professional attainment and tendencies.

I've had the opportunity to experiment with the Karnak Psychic Sensor on the spiritual healer Patricia Pellicciotti, and I can verify by statement of the facts as to the excellence of her faculty, ESK-PK and prognostic.

The graphic reported below is evidence of Patricia's electromagnetic cerebral emissions for every second that she transmitted during a therapeutic healing action at a distance.

You can observe, to the left, that in the mental state of Delta (D) (frequency: 1 Hz), Patricia, while projecting and curing an individual visualized from a distance, produced an elevated visualization of the health problems of the person, sending a frequency of 4.5 Hz, that permitted the reactivation of the psychic and cardio-respiratory functions.

This series of tests reveals and brings to light her primordial or natural state, above all, that in the mental state of Theta (T) she emits an intense action of electromagnetic stimulation. This Theta graph serves to illustrate or bring to evidence her innately developed state, the psychophysical functions (frequency from 4.5 to 7.5 Hz).

There is no doubt about the excellent faculties of spiritual healer Patricia Pellicciotti.

Luciano Muti
Researcher and inventor, Karnak Psychic Sensor

Notes

1 It's believed that prehistoric and Atlantan man had a virtual third eye. The third eye is responsible for human paranormal vision. It was in the middle of the forehead in the position of the pineal gland. Millennia of nonuse of man's natural perceptions closed or deadened it, and now this eye is covered up and atrophied, somewhat in the same way our muscular system behaves from lack of exercise and we lose muscle definition in our bodies.

2 All organic and inorganic substances emit an Aura.

3 Psychometrics is the ability or art of divining information about people or events associated with an object solely by touching or being close to it. Since everything in the universe is vibration, we perceive the vibrations from objects. The accumulation of vibrations occurs as a direct result of the interactions of the individual's Aura with that object. The longer a person has had contact with an object, and the stronger the emotion, the more strongly it becomes charged with the energy patterns characteristic of that person. A clairvoyant can hold the object and become imbued with insights into the individual to whom it belongs.

4 Discovering the true purpose and natural gifts of an individual was the objective of all parents in the ancient traditions. Children of a certain age were presented to the monk astrologers and high priests for the sole purpose of examining their spiritual path. Then, according to what the monks discerned, the children were brought away to the appropriate places of study. This usually occurred about age nine. Discovering our purposes or homework in life is one of the objectives of Aura reading.

5 Mystics, and now laypeople with the aid of the computer, use Aura reading in preventive medicine because it's an unfailing guide to a

person's health. In sound health, the vital rays or forces stream clear and radiate brilliantly; in failing health the color tones are dull and dark, while nebulous spots or patches in an organ's corresponding chakra indicates disease.

6   Neurological science has registered the brain in certain conditions. In moments of rest or relaxation, this altered state is called an *Alpha* brain wave; the state of nervousness intellectual processing is called the *Beta* brain wave. The Alpha state is often referred to as the "dream state." When we are in this altered or Alpha state, the unconscious mind brings about revelations. Other altered states are that of clairvoyants in trance or performing tantric long-distance healing: *Delta* and *Theta*.

7   Tibetans say that these are souls who have been together in previous lives and must come together again for karmic completion. Because of this prior contact of our Auras, we experience a kindred-soul reaction or an Aura familiarity. It's a feeling akin to, "Hey, haven't I met you before?"

8   Ignorance is the root of all disillusions. The ignorances or mental poisons according to Tibetan Tantric medicine are   anger, attachment, avarice, hatred, jealousy, fear, pride, and obtuseness d (close-mindedness).

9   Since vibrations form colors, it's considered to be just an illusion. The best and foremost shamans perceive frequency—not color, as is erroneously articulated in many books about the Aura.

10 This work is possible when the Lha is still attached to our physical body. Otherwise it requires a very special quality of the highest energetic healing realm, such as a shaman's, to work on the cases when the Lha has been stolen or is separating, as in the case of possession or shock, or in the cases of long-term erosion due to infliction of black magic spells.

11 There are many thoughts regarding clothing colors reflecting onto the Aura. Certain colors of the day do indeed have an impact on and change the color of the Aura. Quite often, the novice gets hung up in interchanging the color of the person's clothing for the color of the Aura, but this also becomes evident and influences you less and less with time.

12 The frontal brain regulates will and determination; upper left brain: analysis and calculation; upper right brain: perception, inspiration, creativity; posterior upper brain: magnetism, neuromuscular action.

13 Beta waves occur in electroencephalograms of an adult brain at a frequency of 13-30 cycles per second. In this state we are fully awake, alert, excited, tense. Alpha waves, smooth, regular electrical oscillations, are recorded by the electroencephalograph at a frequency of 3.5-7.5 hertz, the state of deep relaxation, passive awareness, and composure. Theta waves have a frequency of 4-7 hertz and are usually associated with the human intellect, drowsiness, unconscious, and deep tranquility. Delta waves, an even slower type of brain wave having a frequency of 0.5-3.5 hertz, are associated with sleep, an unaware, deep unconsciousness.

14 Since accomplishing spiritual wisdom is a big job, it seems logical that this sageness requires many lifetimes to develop. Therefore, we have many opportunities until we get the message completely fulfilled and purified. It's believed that we are forced into these multiple lives whether we like it or not. There is no free choice as to when we come back, but there is free choice as to whom our parents are. This selection is made according to what we need to do in that lifetime. This gives us the arena for the actual living experiences brought about by being in a certain time and place with a particular set of circumstances. Thus, our environment gives us the chance to work out karma. In esoteric Buddhism, when we have worked out all that karma, we can choose to whom *and* when we return, such as in the case of the highest yogi and lama.

15 This color has a particular type of smoky rather than brilliant aspect, and is darker in the background.

16 In Tibetan tantric medicine, our Lha (Aura) separates at the time of trauma—whether from an accident or other event, even a strong emotional shock such as a divorce, or the improperly mourned death of a loved one. At that time we are more prone to other deep-rooted psychological problems and chronic substance abuse. The consciousness literally ejects away from the physical body and out of the Aura field of the body.

17 When used for healing meditation, the colors that correspond to the chakra/physical body are relative to the predominant color of that chakra; however, all colors are present in each chakra.

18 The wind is the root of all diseases. It's actually called the *wind root*; according to Tibetan psychology, it's *attachment*. Also called the "I"—"I" want it. Example, Mother puts a pacifier in her infant's mouth. Mother creates a sense of attachment; baby responds by

enjoying it; mother takes pacifier out of baby's mouth; baby cries and is unhappy. This unhappiness unfulfilled creates anger. The baby rubs his eyes from frustration, signals anger, then signals confusion: You gave it to me, now you are taking it away." Or, "I want. I got. Now I don't have." Mixed messages, as modern psychologists refer to them, create mental confusion.

19   The physician evaluates the symptoms and causes in three categories: the immediate symptoms (usually those that provoked the patient to visit) and causes, the less immediate symptoms and causes, and the remote symptoms and causes.

20   Karma (an act or deed) is the total effect of a person's actions and conduct during the successive phases of the person's existence, according to the person's destiny and fate.

21   Another similarity and coincidence of concepts in the various philosophies: the new age movement is all pointed toward achieving nirvana through enlightenment. Christianity speaks about heaven. Tibetan Buddhism has enjoyed a high profile, not only in the United States but in all of Europe, during the Aquarian Age, a period of two thousand years during which the influence of Aquarius is prominent. An age lasts for about two thousand years and moves backward through the zodiac. The Age of Aquarius started approximately the time of the new millennium.

22   Black magic is nothing more than perverting positive energies and denigrating them to personal use for selfish motives. What is otherwise possible to do at an extremely high level of altruistic endeavor may also be generated by the minds and level of the user, he who orders it to be done or the operator. In reality, this is what constitutes the difference—manipulating "energy" to heal and energize one's potential creativity for the highest good, or taking and using something that belongs to another, turning it into the users' advantage in a parasitic way. On the other hand, when the power is balanced, a positive shaman can direct thought beams to create great miracles.

23   These cords are referred to as the umbilical cord in other disciplines; it's the same cord, or cords, with which we travel astrally. Ergo, astral projection is only done with our very subtle Lha, and it is reserved only to those with Shaman-trained capabilities. In the first phases of doubling or projecting, you see a silverlike cord connecting two bodies. It's a technique too involved and dangerous to treat lightly

and without preparation. I urge you not to attempt astral projection without the assistance and instruction of an advanced wisdom teacher. Other ordinary beings should travel only with their mind. If you attempt Lha traveling, you risk losing your Lha to lower-level negative spirits as well as larvae that are lying in wait for just these opportunities of limited energy protection.

24   These rituals must be performed on certain days, according to an astrological chart and calculations, based on the person's date of birth. The calculations are based on an Oriental astrology of five elements of the Earth—wood, fire, earth, iron, and water—and then evaluation is made on the strengths and weaknesses of the person, and their good days and their more vulnerable days of the week. This gives us many indications of how and when to proceed.

25   Since Triassic time, rocks, sedimentary deposits, and the system of rocks have evoked curiosity. Gems in particular contain a strong essence or series of vibrations for healing. One of those most mystical is clear quartz. It serves to heal the Aura of those mental and emotional aberrations that can occur with frequencies in a lifetime. Clear quartz has a molecular value to reach larger areas in conditions of negativity that need to be stopped or neutralized. It also works well to open up the *kundalini* (Hindu) or Kalachakra, the doorway to inner and outer power.

26   Tibetan pharmacology uses a number of extraordinary ingredients. Medically, these pills are quite fatiguing to produce. They utilize plants and gemstones; in some cases animals that they need are extinct or protected, such as in the case of rhinoceros. Therefore, of the original 300 pills that they at one time were able to produce, today they can only produce about 160. The effects of Tibetan medicine are very slow but efficacious and permanent. The patients must take the pills for at least three months, minimum. Allopathic medicine, on the other hand, furnishes an immediate symptomatic cure, but most often it does not last long.

About the Author

Reverend Patricia Pellicciotti, an ordained minister, is a spiritual healer, an expert in natural energy therapy and parapsychology.

Sometimes Nature is lavish in bestowing her gifts. This seems to be true of Patricia Pelliccotti who was born with her wisdom tooth apparently fully developed. Her subsequent life and career were simply a play and display of her rare ability of effortlessly knowing without thinking—leading to spontaneous right action. Regressions into previous and present lives (twenty-six total) indicated that she was to do what came naturally in this lifetime as well.

A descendant of Italian female healer potentates, she operates internationally. From the author's early childhood, others began to recognize her paranormal gifts and encouraged research in holistic professions.

As a young professional, Patricia worked on Madison Avenue and Wall Street. She was recognized as a top executive in the financial services industry. Her success rate on behalf of her clients earned her a reputation that was lauded not only by *Who's Who in America, Who's Who in American Women, Who's Who in Finance,* but by the White House and two former presidents. She became famous for applying her intuition and intellect in investment selection and management, and she became a most-sought-after financial and marketing consultant. Her noted special intuitive and problem-solving talents prompted corporations to ask her to advise them on personnel evaluation and recruitment—all by Aura perception.

After an incident that resulted in a near-death experience, she decided to drastically change her professional life to the subtle energetic realm. Her encounters with the Dalai Lama and Tibetan medicine, topped with an irresistible personal call, confirmed her choice.

From that moment forward, applying her renowned problem-solving thumbprint in holistic living issues, she dedicated herself to research of complementary medicine, somatic and folkloric. Soon after, she created a holistic child development and parenting educational system for preschool children—Baby English Playgroup™ and kidology®—with the objective of calling up natural and intrinsic gifts that lie within each individual, spiritually and intellectually.

This knowledge prompted her into establishing a system she calls dolfinology™, a dolphin-human interactive therapy in Cairo, dedicated in particular to children with disabilities and terminal illness.

Patricia is one of the few technical experts in multiple modules and levels of complementary medicine. Thus far, she has expanded her mission to Europe and Arab countries, promulgating amalgamation and research between traditional, natural, and energetic medicine.

Patricia is mostly known in the international arena for her column "Feeling Healthy . . . with Patricia," and her philosophy: auraology® for fun and for real. She appears on radio and television in the United States, Europe, and Egypt, both as a hostess and as a guest, revealing the paranormal and the mysterious.

Other books available by Patricia Pellicciotti
The Happy Face Theory: Indigo Wisdom for Kids and Grown-Ups
Iniziazione alla lettura dell' Aura, l'anima energetic dell'uomo
Convivere Con L'Aura

A personal note from the Author.

Dear Divine reader,

I appreciate your purchase of this book, in particular, because part of the proceeds of all my works are donated to charitable organizations that are dear to my heart.—such as vegetarian/ vegan meal programs for children, worthwhile educational programs for early childhood, etc.

To show our gratitude, upon free registration on our web site, stated your proof of purchase, your will receive a 10% discount on Auraology consultation services.

With respect and love for you who helped us help the children of United States of America,

Patricia M. Pellicciotti
www.auraology.com

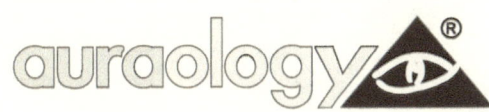

For Fun and for Real